/ / / / / / / / / / / / / / / / / / / / / / /

# THE WOMAN IN THE SURGEON'S BODY

# THE WOMAN IN THE SURGEON'S BODY

## JOAN CASSELL

HARVARD UNIVERSITY PRESS

CAMBRIDGE, MASSACHUSETTS

LONDON, ENGLAND

Copyright © 1998 by Joan Cassell
All rights reserved
Printed in the United States of America
Second printing, 2000

First Harvard University Press paperback edition, 2000

*Library of Congress Cataloging-in-Publication Data*

Cassell, Joan.
The woman in the surgeon's body / Joan Cassell.
    p.    cm.
ISBN 0-674-95467-X (cloth)
ISBN 0-674-00407-8 (paper)
1. Women surgeons.    I. Title.
RD31.5.C38    1998
617'.0232'082—dc21        97-47091

Designed by Gwen Nefsky Frankfeldt

/ / / / / / / / / / / / / / / / / / /

# A(KNOWLEDGMENT$

It is difficult for me to express the depth of my gratitude to the National Endowment for the Humanities, which financed the research on which this book is based. I've always conducted rather dicey anthropological research, which many government agencies and foundations have found theoretically uninteresting or politically suspect (striving to expose the assumed duplicity and venality of powerful groups such as surgeons is more highly regarded in the field of social science than merely studying and attempting to understand them). When I studied the women's movement in the early 1970s, it was considered a bizarre project for an anthropologist. By the time women and feminism became accepted subjects, I was doing something else eccentric: investigating the ethics of social science research. I wrote about children and anthropological research when one's children were considered a purely personal rather than professional issue. When anthropologists realized that the personal *is* professional, I had moved on to study surgeons. I've always had a problem with timing: I was too early to be considered avant-garde, and many people viewed my research as simply peculiar. Of course, this was more than a glitch in timing: I lacked the ability to announce myself with trumpet fanfare as engaged in something remark-able, precedent-shattering, and original. Despite these prob-lems in timing and self-presentation, the NEH funded my original research on general surgeons (Grant RH2051484), the pilot study of women surgeons that showed the project was feasible (NEH Fellowship FB28958), and the research and travel to various sites to complete the study (Grant RH21103-93). Cuts in funding forced me to work in cities where I had friends with whom I could stay. And I paid many of the re-search costs myself. But without the NEH's support, I would not have been able to spend the past fourteen years studying, reflecting, and writing about surgeons.

My thanks to the Rockefeller Foundation Bellagio Study and Conference Center in Italy for a memorable month, in Febru-ary 1996, of soul-nourishing beauty, serenity, and creative stimulation. Freed from the distractions of daily life—and from the temptation to use them as an excuse for not writing—I accomplished far more than I ever thought possible.

For twenty-one years now, Murray Wax has been mentor, colleague, closest companion, and advisor. His loving support has enriched this book and my life.

My thanks to the editors of *American Anthropologist*, who published the essay that became the basis of this book. Their editorial suggestions, along with those of the referees who criticized the manuscript, helped me clarify my thinking and polish my style.

The editors at Harvard University Press helped me to shape and simplify the manuscript. Simple is harder and better than intricate, and I'm grateful for their counsel.

My greatest debt is to the thirty-three women surgeons who allowed an inquisitive anthropologist to trail them through their busy days. Some apparently enjoyed my company; others did not. Several became friends and acted as research collaborators, sharing information and ideas on what it means to be a woman in this martial, male-identified profession. I am also grateful to the women surgeons I corresponded with and those I met at various meetings where I presented my findings; they, too, generously shared ideas and experiences. I have followed anthropological convention and the dictates of confidentiality, altering the names of the women and their colleagues, and disguising various details of their work. (For example, when I describe an incident in which a resident received a scrub suit emblazoned with the words "Slutsky's Slut," her name has been changed but the resident indeed received a scrub suit with an alliterative motto that could be deemed insulting.) Nevertheless, a few of the women may be recognizable. Several are unique, and in such cases concealment is difficult. Whenever I thought that a surgeon might be identifiable, I sent her the relevant section for her approval. The women were generous and deleted very little. I am profoundly grateful to all of them.

/ / / / / / / / / / / / / / / / / / / /

# CONTENTS

# THE WOMAN IN THE SURGEON'S BODY

# 1 / / / / / / / / / / / / / / / / / / / / / / / /

# "WHAT'S AN ANTHROPOLOGIST DOING STUDYING SURGEONS?"

*August 1994: Challenge Posed.* Maureen Barucci had challenged me. She had the temperament of a true surgeon—confident, commanding, competitive—and her unspoken message was remarkably surgical: I'm pretty damn good at what I do—let's see how good you are at what you do.

Dr. Barucci and I had met in 1985, when I was studying general surgeons, and now she was participating in my new research specifically on women surgeons. I had just spent the day with her at Mountainview Hospital, where I had arranged to meet her again the following morning at 7:00. But that night she telephoned to say that the plans had been changed: she would instead be at Southside University Hospital, assisting her partner, Dr. Spector, in a gallbladder removal. She gave driving directions and asked me to meet her in Southside's operating room (OR) at 7:45 A.M. Although I had driven to Southside with her previously, she was aware that I have a defective sense of direction and knew that I might well have difficulty getting to the place on my own.

She had flung down the gauntlet. We both knew it. Could I find the hospital, a good seventy-five minutes from my temporary residence (if I drove like a surgeon, ignoring the speed limits), maneuver my way through the maze of corridors to the locked OR suite, talk my way into it, obtain a clean scrub suit, paper cap, shoe covers, and surgical mask, and locate the room where the procedure would be performed?

I knew a great deal about Dr. Barucci's training to be a surgeon; I had interviewed her about it eight years before. But although she had observed me observing her, she knew little about my own training to study surgeons. This involved more than attending graduate school or learning how to conduct research: the surgeons I studied had trained me to study them.

The anthropologist has been compared to a child: the people she studies must teach her their exotic language and customs. But in a medical setting, one's position is in some ways perhaps closer to that of an inexperienced medical student, who is instructed by nurses, residents, and senior surgeons. In acquiring the language, one assimilates words, grammar, *and* choreography: one masters the appropriate behavior associated with various terms and phrases. Becoming familiar with a new culture involves learning not only what to say but what to *do;* this is so gradual, obvious, and self-evident, that it often goes unnoticed.

*December 1983.* When my study was approved by the hospital's Review Board, I was issued a white lab coat, assigned a locker in the nurses' dressing room, and given a plastic identification card with my name, photograph, department (Surgery), and position ("surgical research"). Belinda, the sole female surgical house officer, took me under her wing. I'll quote from my fieldnotes:

> Belinda . . . showed me how to use the locker and how to dress for an operation . . . I go into the women's locker room, remove

my clothes and white coat and put them in the locker, take a green shirt and pants from the top shelf (where the smallest sizes are). I put them on, then go in through the OR lounge to an anteroom off the lounge, and get paper booties to cover my shoes, a paper hat (rather like a shower cap—there's more than one style, but that's the easiest on the coiffure), and a mask. Then I go out into the OR lounge, through which one goes to get to the OR suite. There's a long corridor, with faucets for scrubbing up, and operating rooms in a row . . . As we walked along the corridor, we could look into the various operating rooms. Things look much gorier [when you're] just peeking in and seeing all that blood . . .

An operation was scheduled for [the chief] for 9:30. One of the nurses explained to me about the "sterile field." Between the instruments . . . and the patient was the sterile field; no one can go into it who is not scrubbed. One could walk on the right, and later, when the instruments on their table were moved to the foot of the patient, one could walk on either side of the patient. If you are not scrubbed, you should stay a foot away from someone who is scrubbed, and always face their front, so you don't accidentally back into them . . . The surgeons were scrubbed . . . (I had a lot of trouble recognizing people I didn't really know well, with all their hair covered, and wearing surgical masks.) . . . The anesthetist (a nurse) was not scrubbed, nor was another nurse ("circulating nurse"), who handed things to the scrubbed nurse ("scrub nurse"). She handed wrapped packages of instruments to the sterile nurse with the first layer unwrapped [and] held out so that the sterile nurse could take [a] package, unwrap it, and put the sterile instruments on her table to hand to the doctors.

The following week, Belinda taught me how to scrub. Again, I'll quote from my fieldnotes:

Very complex and ritualized. First the water, which you put on and off with your knee. The disposable sponge is in a plastic packet over the sink. You clean under your nails with the pick provided for that; throw it in the sink; wash your fingers and hands at least ten times each, including the sides of the fingers . . . Then wash downward from the fingers, with hands held upward so the unsterile portion goes back toward the elbows. You scrub to the elbows—ten minutes, said Belinda. Then, holding your hands in the air, you go into the OR, opening the door with your hip. The scrub nurse hands you a towel. [You use] one end for one hand, the other end for the other hand, making sure it touches nothing else. Then the nurse, or two nurses, put you into a gown and pull the sleeves on. (. . . I made the mistake of pulling the sleeves up with my hands, which made them unsterile, and they had to give me a new gown.) Then gloves are pulled over your hands and over the sleeves of the gown. The gown is fastened in the inside back and on the top by the nurse, who then, holding the belt by a little tab, pulls it around you, so a sterile portion goes over the back; then she tears off the tab she's holding, and you tie the belt with your sterile gloves. Sterile hands must be held above the waist or rested on the operating table—as opposed to unsterile hands, which are held behind one's back.

I never did learn how to scrub properly, but at least I became familiar with the choreography of this crucial surgical ritual. Scrubbing is so significant that surgeons use the term to represent operating. A surgeon will say, "I scrubbed on that case." One "scrubs in" when one enters the OR to assist or operate, and "scrubs out" when removing one's gloves and leaving the room.

*February 1984.* "How's your study going?" inquired the chief resident. "Are you learning what you want to know?" I had been observing general surgeons at this small community hospital for five months now, and I suspect that people were beginning to wonder why I was still hanging around. I told him I was just beginning to learn the language and had yet to reach the stage where I understood not only the words but the music: what people *meant* when they used those words. I mentioned that I had talked with an anthropologist the day before who had studied a group in New Guinea, and she had reported having exactly the same problem. "New Guinea! They eat people there!" exclaimed the resident only half-jokingly. I said nothing, but many of the surgeons I studied seemed as savage, menacing, and alien as any head-hunting tribe.

I spent eighteen months at this hospital, learning to listen to surgeons, understand what they said, and behave properly in various settings. Gradually, I learned to interpret the language of surgeons. I began to understand words, and silences, and was able to laugh at their jokes (an ability to appreciate foreign humor is, some say, a test of when an anthropologist is at home in an alien culture). After studying surgeons at three more hospitals, and observing them at work in thirteen additional hospitals and clinics, I learned that OR suites differed in their geography. Certain features, however, were invariable. One entered the dressing room from a public corridor, and then, wearing clean scrubs, left it from another door that led into the OR suite. Clean scrubs were kept on a shelf in the women's dressing room, and small sizes were often difficult to find. I learned how to "keep sterility" (by avoiding sterile objects, spaces, and scrubbed personnel so that my touch would not contaminate them), and even how to fetch packets when so directed by the scrub nurse, opening them carefully to allow her to remove the contents with her sterile gloves.

After discussing the issue with the first chief of surgery, a reflective and caring man, I decided that patients were under enough stress already and that it would be kinder not to interrupt the proceedings to tell them who I was and what I was up to. I always answered a question with the truth, however, and found that patients invariably seemed delighted that it was not they but the doctors who were the object of scrutiny.

I discovered that surgeons loved challenges—meeting and

issuing them.[1] And they were never so happy as when they were operating: bad temper evaporated, fatigue was forgotten, illness was ignored. Unlike the nurses, who were relieved for coffee breaks, lunch, and the end of their work shift, surgeons kept going until the procedure was finished. (The residents described with relish one procedure, a Whipple, that might take as long as thirteen hours.) The surgeons I studied were arrogant, macho, daring. An attending surgeon in one hospital used to ride to work on his motorcycle through a ghetto area which had suffered a number of violent riots. (This man, who belonged to the Army Reserves, had been in Vietnam during the war; he said he had enjoyed Vietnam but hadn't gotten enough chances to operate.) One day, when he described an incident in which a doctor's car was stoned and its window shattered, I asked whether it wasn't dangerous to ride a motorcycle in that area. "Well, I wear my helmet," he responded (a face-concealing black helmet like Darth Vader's), "and a black leather jacket, and often I wear all black—and I look meaner than they do."

*May 28, 1986.*  Once, when this surgeon, assisted by a surgical Fellow, was scheduled to perform a vascular operation and I jokingly offered to scrub, he took me up on it: for eight hours, two medical students and I held instruments, standing, squatting, and curving our bodies away from the table to get out of the surgeons' way.

> I kept hoping nothing would happen to the patient. If something went wrong and they sued everyone in sight, would I be in trouble? Quite possibly. I would have stayed till the end, I wasn't really all that exhausted (I found it kind of exciting), but I was late for [a friend's] birthday party . . . Dr. Lake had me feel things with the medical students—like a cirrhotic liver, and the graft with the blood running through it. "Feel the thrill!" he

said. "It's astounding!" When I left at 6:15 P.M., a third shift of nurses was starting [the procedure had commenced at 9:30 A.M.]. The first scrub nurse was spelled for lunch. She then left at 2:45, and the woman who spelled her took over. That woman left, and another scrub nurse was just starting at 6:15. The surgeons (and the medical students and me) had not left the room since we scrubbed.

My tension was so great that I had little difficulty emulating the surgeons and going without food, coffee, and bathroom breaks. Being a participant was so exhilarating that I began to understand when surgeons described how, as medical students, they had decided to go into surgery after taking part in a procedure.

*June 1986.* When I finished my study of general surgeons, I understood much, if not all, of their language. Not only had I acquired enough cultural competence to laugh at their jokes, but I was occasionally able to attempt a surgical joke myself. I had learned that surgeons move fast, often vaulting up and down stairs two at a time and racing through mazelike hospital corridors, and I developed the ability to trail them closely so they couldn't give me the slip—as many who did not want to be studied were adept at doing. After observing more than two hundred procedures (ranging from toenail-removals, to amputations, to open-heart surgery) in eight hospitals, I knew how to go into a strange dressing room, find scrubs, change my clothes, and keep sterility in the OR, positioning myself next to the nurse-anesthetist or anesthesiologist and standing on stools to get a view of the proceedings without being underfoot.

I learned more about surgeons as I wrote my book (Cassell 1991), reflecting on my fieldnotes, putting clues together, collating remarks and incidents the surgeons knew would go over my head. Often, it wasn't until I pored over my notes that I perceived certain patterns and realized just what had been going on.

*January 1991.* I had to work out a whole new set of logistics when I began to study women surgeons. There were few women surgeons at each hospital, which meant I had to contact and study each woman individually. As a result, I no longer had my own locker and was forced to devise a complex routine. I stowed my purse in the trunk of my car before meeting the women surgeon at the hospital where she practiced: a purse identified me as an outsider and was difficult to cache in a hospital dressing room. I purchased my own white coat; in the pocket I put my pen and the $3 \times 5$ cards I use for note-taking, and transferred these to the shirt pocket of the scrub suit. I carried a little knapsack, which held sneakers to wear while observing operations, lipstick, and a tiny hairbrush to fluff up my hair when I removed the surgical cap. The knapsack also contained a light lunch suitable for two: women surgeons more often than not skip lunch, so that if I did not want to resort to junk food from coin-operated machines, I found it expedient to bring a few sandwiches and some fruit (explaining that, as a nonsurgeon, I was not trained from an early age to do without food or sleep, and offering to share).

*August 1994: Challenge Met.* Fortunately, following Dr. Barucci's example, I had worn my green Southside Hospital scrub suit home the night before (she told me she always wore "greens," except during office hours). This meant that when I reached the hospital, found a parking place in the garage—at 7:15 A.M. this was not difficult, although my car lacked a doctor's parking sticker—and located the surgical wing, I was wearing greens, sneakers, and my white lab coat. Introducing myself as Dr. Cassell to some surgical residents who were dressed exactly as I was, I asked for Dr. Spector's "lap coli" (laparoscopic cholecystectomy, in which the gallbladder is removed through a small incision with the aid of tiny, long-handled instruments and a miniature camera). I said that I was "observing, not scrubbing," and a resident pointed me in the right direction. The OR suite was locked, but after identifying myself again as Dr. Cassell, I followed someone through the doors. I was found by a helpful Asian woman who seemed to be some sort of supervisor; once more, I introduced myself as Dr. Cassell, telling her I was meeting Dr. Barucci, who was assisting Dr. Spector on his lap coli. She insisted on giving me a locker and key, although I protested that I did not need one. Two nurses showed me where the freshly laundered scrub suits were kept (female nurses shared a dressing room with the female doctors), and I changed from the previous day's greens.

When Dr. Barucci arrived in the dressing room, there I was in clean greens, stowing my possessions in the locker. "Jesus, you're good!" she exclaimed, "It took me years to get a locker. What did you tell them?" "The truth," I responded blandly. In point of fact, I *am* Dr. Cassell, and although it may have taken her years to get a locker, it had taken me even longer to learn how to behave appropriately in this exotic setting. (I subsequently learned that she had obtained permission the day before from the Southside OR supervisor for me to observe; I must admit, however, that I did not know this at the time.)

Dr. Barucci was so fired up by my facility that she decided I would scrub with her and hold retractors. She would thus be able to use both hands to maneuver the miniature camera inside the patient, rather than having to use one hand for the camera and the other for the retractors (the camera displayed Dr. Spector's movements on a large screen that both surgeons watched). If I held retractors I would be unable to take notes, but I let Dr. Barucci direct. I was not unhappy, however, when a nurse objected, appealing to the Asian woman who had given me the locker. The latter said that since I was not a medical student or an attending surgeon at that institution, I could not have hands-on contact with the patient. Consequently, I merely observed and took notes, and was delighted to do so. I am by nature an observer—"voyeur" probably says it even better—which is one reason I became an anthropologist.

*The Question.* I have often been asked what an anthropologist is doing studying surgeons. The most memorable query was posed in 1985, at the second community hospital where I studied general surgeons. Although I routinely went out of my way to introduce myself and ask the surgeon's permission before observing a procedure, this time a nurse on the way into the operating room said, "Joan, you ought to see this." Nothing much was going on in the OR suite, so I snatched a mask, entered the operating room, and moved next to the anesthesiologist, who knew me. The surgeon had just opened the patient. The room was silent as he concentrated on the procedure. Later, however, when the tricky part was over, he looked up and caught my eye: "Who are you?" he inquired in a commanding tone. This was his territory and I was obviously an interloper. "I'm Joan Cassell—I'm an anthropologist studying surgeons," I faltered, knowing I should have introduced myself ahead of time. "Yeah, yeah. Who are you *really?*" he inquired. I repeated my assertion, which he refused to believe. The nurses and anesthesiologist assured him that I truly was an anthropologist who truly was studying surgeons. "What's an anthropologist doing studying surgeons?" he finally demanded. With absolutely no conscious volition on my part, I heard my voice responding: "Well, there were no other primitives left." That surgeon never let me forget this remark. Every time we encountered each other in the hospital, he repeated it with mingled horror and relish.

Perhaps "primitive" was too strong a term, although the phrase delighted the nurses. Surgeons can stage spectacular tantrums and many—the men in particular—occupy a lot of psychic space. A temperamental surgeon can complicate the lives and roil the digestion of subordinates; and nurses, residents, medical students, even secretaries tread cautiously when a prima donna is in full voice.

*More Questions.* Studying general surgeons in the 1980s, I encountered few senior women. I wondered about the women surgeons. Were they also "primitives"—or prima donnas, if you will? What happened when women managed to enter a macho, male-identified profession? Did surgery change the women? Did the women change surgery? In 1986 one of these women related how, in medical school during the Vietnam War, she vowed to do something for her country: after she "got all the tickets" in surgery, she learned to fly and joined the Air National Guard. Discussing differences between men and women, she quoted Kipling: "The female of the species is more deadly than the male." And she said she had heard that the reason cows aren't used in bullfights (they have horns and theoretically could be used) is that the female doesn't close her eyes when she charges! This flight surgeon was surely as macho and martial as any of her male colleagues. Nevertheless, her relations with residents and patients seemed somehow different: softer, more "womanly." Watching her talk to a patient dying of cancer, I observed in my fieldnotes: "She has a lovely manner—warm, compassionate, caring, not smarmy or sentimental." She reported that when she told the patient's wife the surgeons could do nothing for him because his cancer had metastasized, "we cried together." Would a macho male surgeon cry? *Could* a macho male surgeon cry?

This book explores these issues. The research on which it was based inquired whether the women surgeons differed from their male colleagues; if so, how; and whether such differences, if they existed, affected patient care.

*Some Answers.* The answers, like the issues themselves, are complex. I found differences: some of the women differed some of the time from many of their male colleagues. Some did not: they seemed just as macho as the men, if not more so. Unlike male prima donnas, however, who staged some spectacular tantrums when I was present, I observed no female "primitives" throwing fits (although I did hear rumors of explosions occurring when I was absent). But then, the women were given less latitude than the men to indulge in scenes.

I do not resort to biological explanations to illuminate the differences I did find. It's an open question whether men's brains, for example, differ from those of women, and whether such differences might determine or even influence differences in behavior (a cruder version of such explanations was used in the nineteenth century to deny higher education to women). Although I believe gender differences are deep and relatively resistant to change, I am convinced that social factors can explain my findings. To supplement explanations that describe gender as an ongoing social construction, I use the notion of *embodiment*—meaning the way in which people experience and inhabit their bodies, and the way in which these bodies incorporate and express social information. I argue that certain male-identified death-haunted pursuits, such as surgery, test piloting, and race car driving, are *embodied* occupations, and that the body of a woman who aspires to be subject (she who acts) rather than object (she who is acted upon) seems bizarrely out of place to their martial masculine practitioners.

Bodies and what they mean, to those who inhabit and those

who interact with them, are central to my argument. *Although bodies are biological, their meanings are social,* determined from the day of an infant's birth (earlier, if the mother learns the sex of the fetus in utero). These meanings are nonverbal: as French sociologist Pierre Bourdieu says, they are "learned by body." This nonverbal learning endows these meanings with extraordinary power and tenacity. Such embodied knowledge is frequently perceived as biological: a set of self-evident facts based upon indisputable bodily differences. But bodily difference, as research on "intersexed" individuals (those born with anomalous sex organs) in various cultures is demonstrating, is by no means self-evident: the differences that can be observed and those that are inferred may be endowed with any number of cultural meanings. (When studying a female urologist, I sat in on a departmental conference where the fate of an infant born with both male and female sex organs was discussed. It was clear that the decision as to which organs would be kept and which excised, so that the infant would then be defined and reared as male or female, was being made by powerful male surgeons who were following their own social, professional, and cultural agendas. It was also clear that these surgeons conceptualized their decision as indisputably "scientific." It was only the observing anthropologist who perceived the grounds on which it was made as *cultural* and, as such, contestable.)

Anthropological learning, too, is embodied: a new culture is learned in part by body. "Participant observation," a classic anthropological research method, involves such nonverbal body-learning. I assimilated knowledge about surgeons not only through observing them and listening to their conversations, but by learning how to keep sterility in the OR, by scrubbing imperfectly (twice), and by meeting the challenges they issued: from getting myself into an OR suite dressed in fresh scrubs before the surgeon arrived, to holding retractors for eight hours during a vascular operation, to following a sixty-six-year-old woman surgeon up four flight of stairs while responding to her question about interesting recent events in my life (I told her about the tap-dancing lessons I was taking, observing in my fieldnotes: "Challenge posed; challenge met").

Although my argument about embodiment is central to the presentation and explanation of my findings, I believe the findings are absorbing in and of themselves. Naturally, all anthropologists find their data irresistible—but mine really are! Surgery is a sequestered practice, and most of us encounter surgeons at work only when we are naked, horizontal, and unconscious. Women surgeons, who are even scarcer than their male colleagues, are a fascinating group: focused, talented, intelligent, tenacious. This book follows these women as they move through their workdays—holding office hours, making patient rounds, performing operations, teaching students and residents, racing through corridors from one appointment to the next. You will hear them, in their own words, discuss their training and their relations with patients, nurses, secretaries, colleagues, chiefs of surgery, husbands, and children. You will also glimpse me, the observing anthropologist, whose eyes, ears, embodied learning, and theoretical constructs filter all these happenings. Whether or not you agree with my interpretations, I hope you'll find the women as engrossing as I did.

Although I have been studying and writing about surgeons for more than a decade, I do not identify myself as a medical anthropologist. I subscribe to and read medical anthropological journals and try to keep up with at least some of the proliferating writings in the field. I admire and have learned much from the writings of Arthur Kleinman; Byron and Mary Jo Good; Margaret Lock and Nancy Scheper-Hughes on the "mindful body"; Margaret Lock, Deborah Gordon, and others on "biomedicine"; and Emily Martin, whose book title has inspired my own.[2] Recently, much has been published by medical anthropologists on "embodiment." With the exception of Henrietta Moore (1994) and Moira Gatens (1996), neither of whom is a medical anthropologist,[3] few seem to be concerned with the same issues as I.[4]

In the same way, although I think of myself as a feminist and have studied women and, indeed, feminism, I do not define myself as a feminist anthropologist. Again, I read and subscribe to feminist publications, buy, read, and learn from the writings of feminist anthropologists. But, as with the medical anthropologists, I try to keep a certain distance and not get caught up in controversies about "essentialism," "the inequality problematic," feminism versus feminisms, how best to integrate feminist theory and practice, categories of women, and so forth.[5]

In a similar vein, I have carried out almost all of my research in cities in the United States, yet I do not categorize myself as an "Americanist" or an "urban anthropologist."

Perhaps my aversion to such classification is more a matter of temperament than intellectual fealty. I distrust labels and have never belonged to a particular coterie or school. Nor have I kept up with what I think of as the continental flavor-of-the-week: the complex and cerebral thinker, usually French (although Bakhtin filled the role for a while) whom everyone on the competitive intellectual circuit reads, quotes, and relies on for rhetorical flourishes. I study what interests me, using whatever theoretical frameworks or notions seem to explain my findings best. I have never found theories in and of themselves "good to think"; I have subscribed to them only when they seemed to help explain something I was otherwise unable to understand.

I suppose this leaves me in the default category: I am an old-fashioned sociocultural anthropologist, interested in people and what they think, do, and (if it's possible to find out) feel, trying my best to observe and understand whatever I am studying at the time. I write as simply as I can. I address not only anthropologists and feminists, but intelligent nonspecialist readers who are interested in the world at large. I frequently employ what anthropologist James Fernandez calls "an argument of images": I let my descriptions and images carry my argument, allowing readers to draw their own conclusions. Such a style can, on occasion, irritate academics, who may find my work insufficiently theoretical, abstract, or intellectual. The theories are there—but they are often implicit. I want my readers to think for themselves and, if they wish, to disagree with my conclusions.

# 2 / / / / / / / / / / / / / / / / / / / / / / / / /

# BODIES OF DIFFERENCE

*Manliness, manhood, manly courage* . . . there was something ancient, primordial, irresistible about the challenge of this stuff,
no matter what a sophisticated and rational age one might
think he lived in . . . A fighter pilot soon found he wanted to associate only with other fighter pilots. Who else could understand the nature of the little proposition (right stuff / death)
they were all dealing with?

TOM WOLFE, *THE RIGHT STUFF*

When I began studying surgeons in 1983, I was struck
by the martial, masculine ambience of surgery. Several of the
men I interviewed compared themselves to astronauts. The
legendary Chuck Yeager, who emerged unscathed from plane
crashes and became the first man to fly faster than the speed of
sound, might well be the surgeons' heroic ideal. Yeager's char-
acterization of test pilots as "a breed apart" could have been
uttered by a surgeon. The men I studied took the metaphor
of the war on disease literally: from the "front lines" or
"trenches" they carried out "blind maneuvers," attacked "invading tumors," and conducted "search and destroy" missions
(Cassell 1991: 33–59).

Male-identified occupations such as surgeon, test pilot, soldier, firefighter, and race car driver focus on one pole of a set of cultural oppositions: practitioners describe themselves and their comrades as active, strong, decisive, brave, aggressive. "Sometimes in error, never in doubt," is the motto a chief of surgery ascribed to surgeons (Cassell 1991: 37). Symbolic, behavioral, and corporeal meanings are conflated: actors with "the right stuff" perceive themselves as *phallic*.[1]

In each of these vocations, we find ritualized ordeals for initiates, active male bonding, and profound distrust and exclusion of females as participants.[2] And in each, we find the threat of death. What is it about the "ancient, primordial, irresistible" challenge that women would pollute, destroy, negate? What is it about the association Tom Wolfe notes between "the right stuff" and death—about heroism, in short—that makes it something men do *to* and *for*, not *with*, women?[3]

Although men resist their participation on an equal basis, women are essential to these death-haunted vocations: so that they can provide admiration, sex, service, and, perhaps even more important, *so that they can be excluded*—from rituals, knowledge, camaraderie. Such thinking is familiar to anthropologists: the sacred flutes, trumpets, and bullroarers will lose their potency if women learn their mysteries.[4] But without women present to be barred from these mysteries, the secret, as Simmel pointed out (1950: 332), would lose its savor.

Ritualized male development in societies where warlike males are needed and highly valued has been associated with a body of myths and fantasies, which center on what anthropologists term "male parthenogenesis." Adams (1993) discerns a similar theme, which she calls "monosexual male procreation," in the rituals of a Southern all-male military college;[5] and Kaprow (1991: 102) observes that firefighters think of their heroic activities in terms of "giving life." Would the presence of women (as actors, rather than admiring spectators or damsels in distress) in such all-male groups invalidate the "mythic scenario" (Herdt 1981: 277) in which men give birth? Objections to the participation of women in male-identified occupations are always vague; there are no precise words for the devastation that the presence of women would inevitably wreak. Such presence would destroy "morale," "efficiency," "unit cohesion"; or as the president of the senior cadet class of the all-male military college declared, "The very thing that women are seeking would no longer be there" (Adams 1993: 3). A woman's body pollutes and negates the ancient, primordial, irresistible proposition, "the right stuff / death," with its ineffable mythical correlate, "the right stuff / life."

In traditionally male occupations, as in well-documented Amazonian and New Guinean groups where warlike men are glorified, it is commonly believed that the presence of women will destroy the symbolic potency of the concealed rituals and esoteric bodies of knowledge: "The very thing that women are seeking would no longer be there." I suspect, however, that in Western society the causality is reversed and that the very thing (the men believed) women were seeking in surgery, for example, *is* no longer there, or is rapidly vanishing. In other words, women gained entry into the "men's house" when economic and political forces were already in the process of transforming the hypermasculine surgeon-warrior into an endangered and even extinct species. When the surgeon (or the firefighter, or the race car driver) begins to lose his charisma, when his occupation becomes "proletarianized" and he no longer controls his working conditions, when his heroic qualities, his "superhuman strength, courage, or ability," are no longer acknowledged and valued, then the heroes retire or seek new arenas and the opposition to women diminishes.[6] Fewer ambitious men seek to enter the profession, leaving more room for women. As the autonomy, financial rewards,[7] and prestige of surgery diminish, the number of women in the field increases.[8] I believe the two developments are related. As a surgeon's daughter, who was herself a surgeon, remarked: "When the men don't want it any more, they let women into the club."

During thirty-three months of research in the early 1980s, I met only seven female general surgeons above the rank of resident. Although the number of women in general surgery was increasing (Ramos and Feiner 1989: 23–24), I was told of subspecialties where women were actively resisted or barred.[9] I began to wonder what happened when women were admitted into the "men's club." Did the initiates resemble their male peers? Did they display "the right stuff"? Were competent women perceived as pushy and "unfeminine" by traditional, conservative surgeons? Were "feminine" women perceived as incompetent? Did the women undergo a "not entirely benign change"[10] during the course of surgical training, becoming more like the macho, martial, death-haunted men? Or would the participation of women alter certain aspects of surgery?[11]

After finishing my book on general surgeons, I decided to study women in surgery. Literature on women in medicine existed, but I could find no full-scale research on women surgeons.[12] It seemed like a fascinating subject to investigate. At this stage, however, I was not sure whether such research was feasible. To study general surgeons, I had managed to gain entrée into four hospitals. This had been incredibly difficult, as was obtaining enough provisional acceptance to even be able to observe what went on. But once I had managed to pitch my tent in four departments of surgery, I could gather my data, using fairly traditional anthropological methods. I was able to linger in the OR suite, the intensive care unit (ICU), and the surgical wards and observe what went on. There were too few women surgeons in any one hospital, however, to make such a procedure practical for my new study. Even locating the women was arduous. I was unable to discover a central registry listing women surgeons, and names were problematic: there was no knowing whether a "Jesse," "Dale," or "Tenley" was a woman or a man.[13] Because of the scarcity of women surgeons, I did not limit my research to general surgeons but studied every surgical subspecialty I could find.[14]

A fellowship from the National Endowment for the Humanities (NEH) funded a pilot study, during which I worked out the methods. Following the lead of Pearl Katz (1981, 1985; Katz and Kirkland 1988), I had supplemented my study of general surgeons by observing a number of male surgeons individually throughout an entire workday, subsequently administering an open-ended interview to each, which I tape recorded. I adapted this method for studying women surgeons.

The women were located by a combination of networks and serendipity. Each was relatively isolated in her work environment; each knew only one or two female contemporaries who had trained with her, and in many cases these colleagues were practicing in other geographic areas. I was forced to locate and negotiate with each woman on an individual basis. I sent each prospect a letter describing my study, asking if I could spend five days from dawn to dark observing her at work and if I could follow up with a tape-recorded interview.[15] I told her that I would wear a white lab coat, that she was free to introduce me simply as "Dr. Cassell" if she so wished, and that she could bar me from any occasions she wished to keep private.[16] (The five days were generally spread over two weeks, sometimes longer, depending on the surgeon's schedule and my own. The surgeon and I each needed breathing space. I also needed time to type my fieldnotes and recuperate from the surgeons' twelve-to-fourteen-hour days.) The more women surgeons I managed to locate and study, the more prospective contacts I gathered, not only from the women themselves but from colleagues, nurses, and residents; the more women I studied, the easier it became to persuade others to participate.

As with the men, it was difficult to find time in the women's crowded schedules to conduct the interviews (which took anywhere from half an hour to an hour and a half, depending on how communicative, and rushed, each woman was). An accidental development proved fortuitous. One woman and I had dinner together before the interview, and we had such fun that I began to invite each woman surgeon out to dinner as part of the interview procedure. This became a way of thanking her, obtaining a willing participant in the tape-recorded interview, and enjoying what invariably turned out to be a memorable social evening. I allowed each woman to choose the restaurant; and without the fact ever being mentioned, each woman's selection was wonderfully considerate of my limited budget. One woman cooked a delicious dinner for me at her home; the tape-recorded interview was punctuated by the barks of her excited dog, with her voice vainly commanding, "Down, Mozart, down!"

Yet the shift from traditional anthropological methods—the fact that I had to observe each women individually, rather than conducting more centrally located observations of people, sites, and situations over a longer period of time—had significant research implications. Following each woman all day, day after day, I was of necessity associated with her. This obstructed a vital source of anthropological information: gossip. Nurses, residents, and colleagues said little about the surgeon in my hearing, save for compliments when she was liked; at best, a nurse might hint darkly that she knew things which she was certainly not going to tell me. I could not simply hang out in the hospital, to see what developed as a result of various actions and situations. I had to follow each surgeon, often at a dead run or I would lose her. Surgeons move fast, and hospitals are constructed like mazes. Consequently, it was difficult to "triangulate"—to obtain, compare, and weigh different accounts of the same event. Fortunately, in two of the cities where I conducted research, the surgical community was closely knit and my stay was long enough to enable me to hear reports that helped round out and occasionally contradict what I had observed or been told. For example, one surgeon who had a relatively calm manner when I observed her at work was, according to several other doctors, a terror whenever she encountered any sort of ineptitude. A resident reported that she'd once grabbed his lapel, thrust her face in his, and snarled, "What the fuck did you do to my patient!"

Moreover, spending so little time with each woman, I could not enlist people to report events I may have missed. In my earlier study, when a temperamental male surgeon had thrown a screaming tantrum and reduced the head nurse to tears, five different people reported the details to me, including the fact that the head nurse, who I suspected did not particularly like me or my study, had later observed: "Joan Cassell will get a whole chapter in her book on this!" (Although I did not get a chapter on that particular scene, I did get one on the old-time prima donna who caused it.)

When the pilot study was completed, the NEH awarded funds to continue my study at three additional sites.[17] Without this further support, it would have been impossible to publish anything on women surgeons. My pilot study was carried out in an urban area where the surgical community was sufficiently small, and chiefs of surgery and women surgeons were sufficiently scarce, to have allowed a knowledgeable reader to recognize people and settings. Although I observed nothing particularly horrifying, I was told various stories in confidence and found it ethically unacceptable that subjects who were unnamed in my writing might nevertheless be identified. The grant permitted me to study surgeons at different sites, and this made it easier to disguise particulars: the area, actors, and surgical specialties could all be subtly altered to preserve confidentiality. In addition, the geographic diversity ensured that my findings would be somewhat more representative.

I eventually studied thirty-three women in five areas of eastern and midwestern North America (four regions in the United States and one in Canada) who represented fourteen surgical specialties: general surgery (ten women, including one who was trained in plastic, breast, *and* general surgery, and another who was trained in transplant *and* general surgery); breast surgery (six women); plastic surgery (four); pediatric surgery (two); cosmetic surgery with training in otolaryngology, or ear-nose-and-throat surgery (two—these women were trained in ear-nose-and-throat rather than plastic surgery per se, subsequently doing a fellowship in facial plastic surgery); otolaryngology (two); oncology (one, who operated primarily on breasts but also performed various other cancer procedures); hand and nerve surgery (one, who was trained in plastic, hand, and nerve surgery); cardiothoracic surgery (one); orthopedic surgery (one); colorectal surgery (one); urology (one); and neurosurgery (one).

At my first site, I used the medical grapevine to locate senior woman surgeons and chief residents. Eighteen of the twenty-four I contacted agreed to be studied; I spent five to eight working days with each. I found one woman, referred to in this book under the pseudonym "Dr. Elizabeth Bishop," who was so intriguing that I spent extra time observing her (see Chapter 7). At other sites, I made less of an effort to recruit all the women surgeons and concentrated on finding a demographically varied group. If I learned of a surgeon who was African-American or Orthodox Jewish, who practiced a specialty I had not yet observed, or who was in a particularly interesting personal or professional situation, I tried to study her. The resultant "scope sample" thus maximized diversity. I also spent time observing three of the seven women surgeons whom I had observed ten years before, when studying general surgeons. I spent two to five days with each woman, depending on her schedule and my own. At the end of the observation period, I conducted an open-ended tape-recorded interview with thirty-two of the surgeons, inquiring about each woman's medical education and surgical training; having a mentor; being a mentor; views on differences between men and women surgeons; relationships with superiors, colleagues, and subordinates; and how she reconciled the demands of surgery and private life.

Unsurprisingly, given the fact that the profession has only recently begun opening up to both sexes, the women who participated in the study tended to be young. Ten were aged 30–35, twelve were 36–40, seven were 41–45, one was in the 46–50 range, one in the 56–60 range, one in the 61—65 range, and one in the 66–70 range. Following is a more precise breakdown:

| Age at time of study | Number of women |
| --- | --- |
| 30 | 2 |
| 32 | 3 |
| 33 | 1 |
| 34 | 3 |
| 35 | 1 |
| 37 | 4 |
| 38 | 3 |
| 39 | 1 |
| 40 | 4 |

| Age at time of study | Number of women |
|:---:|:---:|
| 41 | 2 |
| 42 | 3 |
| 44 | 1 |
| 45 | 1 |
| 46 | 1 |
| 59 | 1 |
| 62 | 1 |
| 66 | 1 |

The marital and family situations of the women differed. Twenty-one were childless; of these, twelve had never married, two were divorced, and seven were married. Of the remaining women, all of whom were married, four had one child, two had two children, three had three children, and three had four children.

More than half the participants in the study (seventeen) had been practicing for fewer than 6 years. Eight had been practicing for 6–10 years, four for 11–20 years, one for 21–30 years, and two for more than 30 years. Following are the exact numbers:

| Years in practice | Number of women |
|:---:|:---:|
| Chief resident | 5 |
| 1 | 5 |
| 2 | 1 |
| 3 | 4 |
| 4 | 1 |
| 5 | 1 |
| 6 | 1 |
| 7 | 2 |
| 8 | 2 |
| 9 | 2 |
| 10 | 1 |
| 11 | 2 |

| | |
|---|---|
| 12 | 1 |
| 13 | 1 |
| 28 | 1 |
| 32 | 1 |
| 34 | 1 |

One woman declined to be interviewed, but I was able to obtain some information about her from a colleague who had trained with her. Consequently, the sample size for some categories of data is thirty-three, while for others it is thirty-two.

*The Relationship of Observer to Observed.* Anthropologists and sociologists have traditionally studied peoples with less power than they. Although much advice has been given, over the years, to "study up" (see, for example, Nader 1969), until relatively recently anthropologists have tended to concentrate on "exotic peoples," and sociologists have preferred to study "nuts, sluts, and preverts" rather than people similar to themselves.[18] The structural and social asymmetry of such research has generated a literature of ethical and political injunctions, directing investigators to respect, consult, and collaborate with those studied. The traditional anthropological term "informant," meaning an indigenous helper who explains local customs, concepts, and phrases, has been jettisoned in favor of "consultant," which more fully expresses the desired relationship between researcher and researched. Somewhat more recently, interest in the work of various continental theorists has generated a desire to create a "dialogue" between the person who studies and those who are studied.

I have taken little part in these debates because, with the exception of a summer in the West Indies learning to "do" fieldwork (Cassell 1987), I have been unable to conduct traditional anthropological research. I was married and the mother of two young children at the time I was working on my Ph.D. The family was not transplantable, so in the early 1970s, rather than traveling to some exotic site to conduct traditional dissertation fieldwork, I somewhat reluctantly formulated a research project in the city where I lived. And rather than concentrating on traditional anthropological subjects in an urban milieu, I focused on a theme suggested by my male advisor as a joke: the women's movement in the United States. The social class, dress, language, and background of the women I studied were very similar to my own. I even conducted research in my own university community, joining a campus women's liberation group, leafleting near the subway station, participating in demonstrations, and serving as a member of a delegation that confronted the university president. It was nerve-racking: nothing in my training had prepared me for this. The women I studied were part of the audience for my dissertation and subsequent book, *A Group Called Women: Sisterhood and Symbolism in the Feminist Movement* (1977). This generated much reflection, and I learned a lot about what an anthropologist owes the people she studies and about the ethics of revealing and concealing (Cassell 1977b, 1978). After studying the ethical problems of social research,[19] a topic stimulated by my unconventional dissertation work, I began my study of surgeons.

In the early 1980s, I knew of few anthropologists who were conducting research on Western doctors.[20] Again, I was doing something relatively far from the mainstream, not because I am all that unorthodox but because the subject presented itself and appeared interesting, and I decided to go for it. In conducting this research, I was probably "studying up." I say "probably" because at that time I was married to a doctor, was more or less the same age as the senior men I studied, and was in some ways treated by them as a doctor's wife. When these men talked down to me (and the surgeons frequently did talk down to nonsurgeons), I *felt* like an equal, whatever their perceptions of me might have been. But our relationship was asymmetrical. The surgeons did *not* want to be studied. Malpractice suits and insurance premiums were escalating, the climate was becoming increasingly inimical to doctors, and, as a group, the surgeons saw no advantage and many possible disadvantages to having a social scientist observe them at work. This was compounded by the topic of my NEH-funded study: moral self-regulation in surgery.[21] Without my husband's connections—including a medical school classmate who was a chief of surgery, a remarkable man who hoped my findings would benefit the profession—I never could have gained entrée. Once in, I felt I had to emphasize my identity as a doctor's wife, and to play up my small physical stature, soft voice, and unthreatening demeanor as a female who admired and looked up to the heroic surgeons I was studying. I *was* a small, soft-spoken doctor's wife and I *did* admire many if not all of the men, but still there was a certain amount of exaggeration if not outright deception in my stance. Anthropological fieldwork is taxing, but studying general surgeons was even more arduous. Almost every night, I returned home discouraged and emotionally drained.

Studying women surgeons almost ten years later was different. Much of the time it was an absolute delight. Ethnographic research always involves hard work: the researcher must focus her attention, take in as much as possible, scribble brief notes without losing the flow of conversation and activities, behave in some ways like a recording instrument while at the same time interacting like a social being. The surgeons worked long days and covered a lot of ground. They had been trained in endurance from Day One; those who could not stay the course dropped out to enter less taxing specialties. Nevertheless, the research situation and relationships were far more comfortable in the later study, requiring far less social and emotional effort. With many of the women surgeons, I achieved the ideal research relationship: they became collaborators, as interested as I in the issues under investigation. They too wanted to know whether and how they differed from the men; they too were interested in the concepts of "doing gender" and in hearing (and exchanging) descriptions of the pressure I observed being exerted on them to behave in "feminine" ways. I played my cards less close to my chest. Perhaps because I was older and had more research experience than in my earlier study, or perhaps because of the comfortable relationships the women and I so frequently fell into, I was as open with them as I hoped they would be with me. Several displayed tremendous empathy and thoughtfulness.[22] There was a feeling of parity, of a collective "we," as opposed to the male surgeons, where I was studying "them."

I do not wish to suggest that I was in a kind of ethnographic Eden, conducting research amid a choir of admiring and helpful surgeons. Two of the women who had given permission for me to study them ended up behaving as though they did not particularly like me, eluding me in hospital corridors and avoiding conversations. Another, after agreeing to participate in the project, set up all sorts of last-minute barriers, complications, and difficulties after I arrived in her city, with limited time and several days set aside specifically to study her. (In the course of one afternoon, the same woman changed her mind six times as to whether she was free to respond to my questionnaire and then dine with me. Eventually, she agreed to have coffee; but after we had consumed a first course at a coffeehouse, this segued into an enjoyable dinner.) The women sometimes experienced events and situations that they wished to conceal from me: I could sense they were keeping secrets but could not determine their content, and this made for a certain discomfort. I had discouraging days. But the sense of despair I had felt when studying the men—the feeling that there was no way I could successfully complete my project—was absent. Instead I felt excitement and occasionally exhilaration. Several women became friends whom I still visit. Two women requested my help. One was faced with a possible malpractice suit: a patient whom I had observed her examine and talk with was contending that the surgeon had not explained the risks of a particular procedure. I sent the surgeon the relevant notes for that day, containing descriptions of her meticulous explanations. The second was involved in an acrimonious divorce and custody fight that erupted after my research; she wondered if I had made notes on various interactions I had observed between herself, her husband, and her children. I had indeed, and sent her lawyer the notes. There has been much discussion of reciprocity, of how anthropologists can thank those who allow them into their lives; this is the first research situation in which I have been able to reciprocate so directly.

## EMBODIED DIFFERENCE

I have heard surgeons declare that surgery is a "body contact sport."[23] The phrase refers to more than the proverbial aggressiveness and intrepidity of surgeons. It indicates that, as a medical specialty, surgery is uniquely physical, distinctively embodied. Surgery involves bodies—those of surgeons as well as of patients. During an operation the body of the surgeon makes brutal contact with the body of the patient, piercing the envelope of skin, assaulting the flesh, violating bodily integrity. The patient's body is irreversibly altered.

Western medicine deals with bodies.[24] In medicine, "much of clinical and practical knowledge is 'embodied' knowledge—knowledge sensed through and with the body. This includes senses of sight, sound, touch, smell" (D. R. Gordon 1988: 269). Some specialties, however, are more embodied than others. Fundamental to being a surgeon is physical proficiency, or "good hands" (Cassell 1991: 11–12); like sports and the performing arts, surgery is based on *body* learning, *body* knowledge.[25] The Japanese phrase *karada te oboeru*—"learning or remembering through the body"—refers to such tutelage.[26] One masters these skills by doing, not talking. The extent of embodiment seems roughly parallel to the prestige system among doctors: psychiatrists are on the lowest rung ("They're not real doctors," an internist sneered),[27] while at the other end surgeons loftily disdain the less embodied specialties. I remember a surgical house officer who referred to "medical doctors" as "fleas" (see Konner 1987: 383), and a surgeon I studied said of an internist, who in her opinion gave dangerously poor care, "Hold him down while I drive a stake through his heart!"[28]

Every medical specialty prizes clinical knowledge that is "sensed through and with the body," but surgery makes unique use of "sight, sound, touch, smell." Surgeons' eyes, hands, and instruments probe the hidden recesses of patients' bodies. Bodily discharges assault their senses: bloody jets, noxious smells, stomach-turning effluvia. Only half-jokingly, an ear-nose-and-throat specialist told me that surgical subspecialties are chosen by the secretions a candidate cannot tolerate: "I hate shit," she declared, "but I don't mind snot."

What does it mean when the body of the surgeon—the intrusive gazer, the violator, the recipient of sensory assaults—is that of a woman? Does the woman in the body relate to the bodies of patients the same way that a man would? Does her body have the same meaning to patients, colleagues, superiors, subordinates? And if the woman in the surgeon's body indeed behaves differently, relates differently, and is perceived differently, how can we understand such differences? Conversely, how can we understand similarities?

When I began a pilot study of women surgeons in 1991, I was interested in difference. I wanted to know whether women surgeons differed from the general surgeons I had observed at work almost ten years earlier, who were predominantly men (Cassell 1991). I wondered whether the women surgeons were as arrogant, daring, and warlike as their male colleagues and, if so, whether they were punished by their co-workers for such "unfeminine" qualities.

My early observations were contradictory, and I had difficulty finding a theoretical framework that would illuminate what was going on. Planning my inquiry, I was influenced by thinkers who emphasize *differences* between men and women. Then, while conducting fieldwork, I was introduced to the writings of anthropologists and sociologists who discuss "doing" or "negotiating" gender: rather than examining gender differences as such, these theorists focus on the *social construction* of such differences. And finally, after completing my research, I read and reread the work of scholars who discuss the *embodied* nature of experience, identity, and gender.

A scene from my fieldnotes will illustrate the explanatory power of these theoretical approaches. It's important to note that what must be explained is not a *single incident*, which may be interpreted various ways, but a *pattern of events*. Nevertheless, the scene will shed light on the way in which my observations related to the explanations I found most helpful.

A pediatric surgeon in her late sixties is conducting office hours at a university hospital for children. The walls of the examining rooms and hallways are covered with children's drawings, which look cheerful and attractive. (In the adjoining wing, a senior male pediatric surgeon is also holding office hours; his walls are bare.)

> With the first girl, who was about ten or so, she looked at her musical-note earrings and asked if she liked music . . . With the next infant, she lifted him high in the air and said admiringly, "What a handsome beast!" He was, too. She tickled him till he smiled, and then, while explaining what was going on, she kept stroking the baby's tummy and then hair, lovingly . . . To one kid she said, after doing something minor, "You're a great patient, probably the best patient I'll see today!" When she went into a room where a boy was looking glum, she said, "Are you unhappy? Or afraid?" She kept on talking to him about what would happen to him when he was operated on [a tonsillectomy], till she got to the "popsicles" there for him, at which he cracked a smile. Then she teased him about his stylish jeans jacket being too big for him. By the time he and his mother left, the atmosphere was very relaxed. With one baby, as she talked to the parents, she played with the baby's hand. The examining table was covered with disposable paper, and each room had crayons . . . (With one mother, who needed a particular kind of scissors to care for her child's bandages, she said, "Oh just take these—it's the best way to get them.") When told about one kid waiting for her, she said, in a joyful tone, "Oh, Gregory! My favorite patient!" To Gregory's mother she said, while talking to her, "You're a good mother!" and seemed to mean it. The mother told [the surgeon] how she's going to social work school to get a master's in social work, and how much she'd like to do a practicum at [the children's hospital]. When [she was] dictating her notes, I heard [the surgeon] put in that the mother was going to social work school and wanted to do a practicum there, and that they should try to get her, since she has experience (with sick kids). When she came into another room, she said (truthfully), "I heard there was a cute baby in here!" She said to the older woman there with the parents, "Grandma?" The grandmother assented, and [the surgeon] asked, "How many grandchildren?

Boys or girls?" She asked the mother, "This your first? What's the other?" And she listened to the responses.

The nurturant, "womanly," "maternal" manner in which this unmarried, childless surgeon interacted with patients and families was similar, in many ways, to that of another pediatric surgeon I observed who is married and has four children. Here's a brief glimpse of the second woman during office hours:

> To one frightened boy of about seven, who didn't want her to close a deep cut on his chin with steristrips and who was weeping, yelling, and wriggling, she said, "Baby doll, I'll do it with you standing up!" I suspect she talks to them the way she does to her own kids. Afterward, she told him how great he had been. In each case, she asks them the questions she thinks they may be able to answer: "Are you reasonably healthy?" "Have you had any other operations?" She clearly likes and enjoys kids, and it shows.

To my surprise, both surgeons, when interviewed, denied that the way women surgeons relate to patients and families is different from that of men. Although the younger woman had once told me that women had something special to bring to surgery, during the interview she denied that women behave differently from men. When I questioned the older woman about differences between male and female residents, she said: "I've had women residents come through here that are very abrupt. I've had some guys come through here that are just fantastic."

The questions I asked these two surgeons have been much discussed in recent years. Psychologists, sociologists, biologists, and philosophers have debated whether women and men are fundamentally different or essentially the same.[29] Sociobiologists, convinced that anatomy, biology, and genetics are destiny, maintain that women are "naturally" smaller and weaker, and less gifted spatially, mathematically, and analytically.[30] Doubtless they would argue that the nurturant behavior of the two pediatric surgeons described above was biologically based, perhaps selected for during the evolution of *Homo sapiens*, allowing more children of "maternal" women to survive and pass on their genes. Their explanation—only slightly simplified—might be characterized as: men hunt, fight, and make war, whereas women nurture and rear children; these behaviors are encoded in the brain or genes, allowing for reproductive success. If nurturance is biologically female, however, why are some women surgical residents "very abrupt" with patients and families, and some men "just fantastic"? And why did the two pediatric surgeons themselves assert that differences in caring and compassion cannot be associated with gender?

It is difficult to determine whether significant genetic or neurological differences between men and women exist, and nearly impossible to discover whether such contrasts, if they do exist, stimulate disparate behavior in men and women. (How could one design an experiment with humans to tease out the biological, social, and psychological variables?) As a social scientist, admittedly prejudiced against such biological determinism (which sounds uncomfortably close to Calvinist predestination), I am convinced there must be a simpler and more convincing explanation for this scene and others I observed.[31]

Sociobiological determinists divide humans into two groups: men are hunters, women are nurturers.[32] Similar contrasting oppositions are found in the writings of a number of feminist psychologists, sociologists, and philosophers.[33] Whether such contrasts are attributed to developmental experiences, "maternal thinking" (Ruddick 1989), or cultural imperatives, these "difference theorists" argue that women are, or tend to be, more nurturant, caring, and cooperative than men, who are more independent, detached, and hierarchical. Both biological determinists and difference theorists find *essential differences* between women and men.[34]

The two pediatric surgeons I have described were indeed remarkably nurturant and caring with patients and their families. The older woman, however, cannot be characterized as particularly gentle, feminine, or cooperative: in many ways, she was a pretty tough cookie. I cannot picture this surgeon ever having allowed herself to be relegated to the cave with the women and children, while the men brandished clubs and hurled challenges at one another. One day, I observed her settle a wager with a young male surgeon, as to who could crouch longer with knees bent, back against the wall; this sixty-six-year-old woman "sat" against the wall for thirty-five seconds, with the nurses and residents timing her. The same day, while going up the stairs two at a time, from her office to the OR, she told me she was preparing for a skiing vacation. At first, I thought she'd said "skating vacation," but she told me no, you might break your arm skating. "Skiing isn't known for being healthy either, is it?" I asked. Well, she replied, if you break a leg, you can usually still manage to operate.

In my pilot study, I observed that some women surgeons differed from their male colleagues in some ways some of the time; others differed in other ways at other times; and some displayed more similarities to their aggressive, macho male peers than they did differences. Thus, a woman who seemed to be compassionate with patients might be cold and commanding with nurses; another, who seemed gentle and noncompetitive with patients and subordinates, might go to the mat with the chief of surgery in a battle about her salary; yet another might be abrupt with patients, competitive with peers, and hard on subordinates. Contrasts between women's perspectives, values, and behavior and those of men just did not explain my complex and ambiguous findings.

I then turned to a more recent body of theory and research which analyzes gender as a "negotiated" or "constructed" category.[35] Gender, in this view, does not exist in and of itself; instead, it is *produced* during interaction.[36] Rather than examining differences, scholars who subscribe to this theory explore the *social construction* of such differences. In this approach, gender is something that is not possessed but *performed:* one does not *have* a gender—one *does* gender. Rather than being fixed, "natural," and innate, gender is seen as a process or "category of difference" that can be negotiated, resisted, altered.[37]

The two pediatric surgeons, then, when they related to patients and families in a motherly fashion, could be perceived as "doing gender." They were acting as they and those around them expected women in our culture to act. One advantage of this "social constructionist" approach is that the anthropologist can concentrate on observed behavior, rather than searching for "deep structure" and speculating about what each surgeon is "really" like.

The notion of doing or negotiating gender helped explain many of my findings. Conducting research, I observed exchanges between women surgeons and patients, nurses, chiefs of surgery, colleagues, and residents in which "feminine" behavior was elicited, encouraged, even extorted, at the same time that aggressive, "masculine" displays were penalized. It was obvious that, if the women surgeons' behavior was not entirely socially constructed, it was surely influenced by interaction with the people around them.

Nevertheless, as I continued studying surgeons, I found there was something unsatisfying about the social constructionist approach. It explained much, yet too often these theorists discussed women as though they were a collection of disembodied "discourses," "behaviors," "attitudes," "values," "processes," and "categories." Moreover, the view of gender as a process based solely on interaction seemed at odds with the depth and persistence of the gender-related incidents I was observing, not only in those who exacted "appropriate" behavior from the women, but in the women surgeons themselves. Gender may well be affected and shaped by interaction, but there is more to it than interaction and performance. I observed too many gut reactions related to gender (male surgeons enraged by women invading their precincts; women who behaved in "feminine" fashion when the interactional situation called for raw aggression) to be able to ascribe these incidents solely to superficial and easily eradicated sources.[38] I also observed distinct limits to the negotiation of gender—limits which apparently varied, depending on ethnicity, geographic region, and social class. There was something else going on, something profound, nonlogical, and nonverbal: something *embodied*.

Disembodied discussion of the social construction of difference ignores the depth, persistence, and power of difference. If we wish to understand it thoroughly, we must explore the embodied nature of identity and experience. For this, I shall make use of Pierre Bourdieu's concept of habitus.[39] "Habitus" might briefly be defined as *embodied social structure* which is passed on from generation to generation. The habitus shapes the body; at the same time, the body expresses the habitus. Habitus is not something that you *think* but is something that you *are*, and what you are is based on what you *do*, on the actions and reactions of your body. The habitus is composed by activity through time, rather than by abstract structures or ideas. Social structure and practice are expressed in and by the body. Henrietta Moore, who speaks of "lived anatomy," observes: "Praxis is not simply about learning cultural rules by rote; it is about coming to an understanding of social distinctions through your body, and recognizing that your orientation in the world, your intellectual rationalizations, will always be based on that incorporated knowledge" (1994: 78).

The bearing, size, shape, and movement of the body symbolize, express, and reinforce basic social divisions.[40] This incorporated knowledge is below the level of words, in possessor and observer. I am convinced that habitus explains the "intuitive," "tacit" cultural knowledge we have about those we meet: the way people stand, dress, move, act, react, and physically interact communicates wordlessly their social and sexual location and self-image. I came to know a lot about the women surgeons in a relatively brief time. I did not always know, however, just what it was that I knew. One's body may know things about another body that never achieve conscious, verbal expression.[41] Illustrating such nonverbal knowledge, in terms of "body schemas" associated with different social classes, Bourdieu presents a stunning juxtaposition of two photographs (1984: 210): first, a working-class body-builder in a pair of scanty trunks, flexing his well-oiled muscles; second, the aristocratic president of France, Valéry Giscard d'Estaing, in tennis whites, gracefully swinging his racquet. One glance and the social class of each body is evident, even to an American unfamiliar with the nuances of French class distinctions.

In a passage that might well refer to the embodied anxiety of men who cannot tolerate a woman's body in their intrepid, male-identified, embodied occupations, Bourdieu notes:

> The ultimate values, as they are called, are never anything other than the primary primitive dispositions of the body, "visceral" tastes and distastes, in which the group's most vital interests are embedded . . . The sense of distinction . . . which demands that certain things be brought together and others kept apart . . . re-

sponds with visceral, murderous horror, absolute disgust, meta-physical fury, to everything which lies within Plato's "hybrid zone," everything which passes understanding, that is, the embodied taxonomy, which, by challenging the principles of the incarnate social order, especially the socially constituted principles of the sexual division of labour and the division of sexual labour, violates the mental order, scandalously flouting common sense. (1984: 474–475)

The term "sexism" is too abstract, too *disembodied*, to describe such a visceral rejection of the wrong body in the wrong place; perhaps "misogyny" is more accurate. Thus, after one of the U.S. Navy's first female fighter pilots died in a plane crash (*New York Times*, October 30, 1994: A33), several news organizations in southern California received faxes—apparently from what the *Times* described as "disgruntled" male aviators—suggesting that she crashed because she was incompetent. If indeed these were sent by male pilots, the term "disgruntled" does not adequately represent the emotions of such ferocious exemplars of "the right stuff": their visceral, murderous horror, their absolute disgust, their metaphysical fury on seeing a woman's body at the controls of a fighter plane. (I suspect that similar visceral, murderous horror motivated the cadets who tried to set their female peers on fire—the first women to be admitted to the Citadel military academy.)

Women surgeons have described similar reactions from male colleagues, but I have few such examples. Perhaps few incidents occurred—or perhaps it is easier for a woman surgeon to cope by "forgetting" such events. After spending time with a woman who related a number of misogynistic episodes (see Chapter 8), I recounted some to surgeons who had become friends of mine in the course of the study; each quietly indicated that she, too, had been exposed to similar behavior. Although I had asked a number of probing questions while conducting my research, the incidents did not come to light until elicited by the stories.

Resistance to the presence of women is generally subtler. One woman told how, during her surgical training, she finally realized what it was that disturbed her about the way the male surgeons treated her. "They'd worked it out," she said, describing the men's attitude toward women surgeons. "Either you're not a woman—you're a bear, a dog, or a lesbian. Or you're not a surgeon—you're no good." Her analysis illuminated the stories of two other women: each stated that, during her surgical training, a senior man had advised her to always wear lipstick so that no one would assume she was a lesbian. One of the women recalled that, as a medical student on a surgical rotation, whenever she'd been summoned to the emergency room in the middle of the night, the older female resident would remind her: "Oh, we have to put lipstick on!" The other woman, the first female admitted to an elite surgical training program, always kept some handy so that she could wear it when she was in her scrub suit—a fact whose significance was underscored by her chief of surgery, who wanted to know if she'd shown the lipstick to me. "She noticed it herself," the woman replied.

Women who possess the wrong body in the wrong place can't be "real" women if they've placed themselves in that situation ("You're not a woman—you're a bear, a dog, or a lesbian"). Hence the lipstick, as embodied refutation of *not-woman* status. The male mentors, who counsel the women to wear lipstick, also advise them on becoming proficient surgeons ("Or you're not a surgeon—you're no good"). The wrong body, but the right place: the body can move, react, think, behave like a surgeon. Each half of the double accusation—wrong body, wrong place—must be rebutted. Thus, a *New York Times* op-ed piece on the Navy fighter pilot who crashed in 1994 (November 2: A23) emphasized both her beauty and her competitive blood-lust (her radio call signal was "Fang," from a remark she made to a reporter about how women could equal men in ferocity: "Why not? My fangs grow as long as anybody else's"). Both parts of the accusation have been addressed: the body belongs to a "real" woman, yet in its aggressiveness it resembles those of the male "jet jocks." The reporter noted the woman's physical beauty (an embodied argument), and the pilot, rather than describing herself as "ferocious," referred to her "fangs" (another embodied argument).

The women who took pains to wear lipstick were residents and a medical student. In the sexually polarized world of surgeons, it is advantageous for a female trainee to be perceived as a "real" woman, rather than something that lies within "Plato's hybrid zone," violating the "incorrigible proposition" (Kessler and McKenna 1978) that humans are naturally divided into two, and only two, genders. A lone female resident may be "adopted" by a male chief of surgery as a symbolic daughter; his protection eases the social and psychic rigors of training, mitigating onslaughts by peers and senior surgeons. Thus, the chief resident whose lipstick was pointed out by her chief said that when she had entered the program as its first woman, the chief, Dr. Slutsky, had given her a scrub suit with "Trauma Momma" and "Slutsky's Slut" emblazoned in red on the back. From the way she related the story, it was apparent that she had met the challenge posed by these terms by taking it for granted that they were affectionate nicknames, which they then became. One day in the OR, after she had accomplished a particularly difficult maneuver, a senior surgeon said, smiling broadly, obviously quoting someone else: "That's mah slut!" He continued, "I've been waiting for a chance to say that!" Learning that this was the chief's phrase, a medical student, assisting at the procedure, asserted: "That's harassment!"

"No, no, no, no," said the young woman, "He was a sup-porter!" I once observed the chief, who was at least 6'5", stand over this small, slender woman and address her in an explo-sive, threatening tone: "Do that or you're dead meat!" On an-other occasion, he said: "Starting day after tomorrow, you be-long to me. You belong entirely to me!" When I ventured, "You sound like King Kong holding the woman in his hand," he responded darkly, "It's worse than King Kong." As he uttered what sounded like horrendous threats, she smiled up at him, unfazed; it became clear that this woman, who came from a family of girls, and the chief, who had five daughters, had a perfect understanding. Had she lacked stamina or surgical proficiency, she would not have been accepted by the chief. Nevertheless, this woman's ability to say and do the right thing in response to his challenges seemed to me to be based not upon thinking or calculation but upon a kind of intuitive, embodied understanding.

I have observed the same chiefs of surgery who adopt young residents as symbolic daughters direct savage attacks against female peers, whose experience, knowledge, competence, and demeanor do not elicit fatherly warmth. Such responses, I sus-pect, involve "visceral tastes and distastes," and the men themselves might have difficulty explaining what they are do-ing and why. Unlike the abstract intellectual arguments they might offer after the fact to justify such gut reactions, these "primitive dispositions of the body" are anterior to "pure" reason, and all the more powerful for this reason. Bourdieu notes that "the principles em-bodied in this way are placed beyond the grasp of consciousness, and hence cannot be touched by voluntary deliberate transformation, cannot even be made explicit; nothing seems more ineffable, more incom-municable, more inimitable, and therefore more precious, than the values given body, made body" (1977: 94).

Values given body, made body, are inculcated very early: before acquiring the mother language, the mother's language, the child comes to know the mother's body language. It is an individual's earliest upbringing that establishes the habitus. Beginning in infancy, the movements of bodies in physical space are suffused with social meanings and values, so that movements in physical space and those in social space are sensed as equivalent. This is "practical knowledge," body knowledge, independent of thought.

Such practical body knowledge is, I believe, what the scientist-philosopher Michael Polanyi is referring to when he discusses "tacit knowledge," indicating that "we can know more than we can tell" and stating that "the transmission of knowledge from one generation to the other must be predominantly tacit" (1967: 61). The examples Polanyi gives for tacit knowing all involve embodied knowledge: one can recognize someone's face without being able to say how this is done; experimental subjects who are given electric shocks when certain words are uttered will subsequently avoid these words, yet are not aware that they are doing so. "Our body is the ultimate instrument of all our external knowledge, whether intellectual or practical," he asserts (1967: 15).

Polanyi is addressing the tacit knowledge that generates scientific discovery. Philosopher Moira Gatens, in contrast, refers more specifically to the embodied, wordless knowledge of what it means to be a woman or man in a particular social setting. She argues that in every culture bodily experiences and events are endowed with essential meanings, which are often unconscious; as a result, complex and pervasive networks of images, symbols, and signification link the male body with masculinity and the female body with femininity. She suggests that "some bodily experiences and events, though lacking any *fixed* significance, are likely, in all social structures, to be privileged sites of significance . . . For example, menstruation is likely to be one of these privileged sites. The fact that menstruation occurs only in (normal) female bodies is of considerable import." She continues: "Given that in this society there is a network of relations obtaining between femininity and femaleness, that is, between the female *body* and femininity, then there must be a qualitative difference between the kind of femininity 'lived' by women and that 'lived' by men" (1996: 9).[42]

Let us return to the two pediatric surgeons conducting office hours. If we interpret the way they relate to their patients as based on *embodied knowledge* of the various images, symbols, and meanings of being a woman in our culture, then we should not be surprised that their interactions are "feminine" and nurturant. These women have incorporated maternal behavior from the first moment they were snuggled by their mothers. As little girls, they were wordlessly shown how to nurture their baby dolls—behavior that was very different from the way little boys are encouraged to play with their warlike dolls. They learned to express tenderness toward younger children in a particular fashion, similar to the way their mothers expressed tenderness to them—as opposed to how little boys learn to express comparable interest in babies and little children, which is likely to resemble the playful, mock-challenging manner their fathers adopted with them. This is practical, tacit body knowledge, for which there are few if any words. "What is 'learned by body' is not something that one has, like knowledge that can be brandished, but something that one is" (Bourdieu 1990a: 73). The "lived anatomy" of these women, their embodied principles, values, and ways of acting, are so much a part of them that the women are unaware of it. Since they may not be conscious of what they are doing and why, the two surgeons may well deny that women differ from men in the way they relate to patients. Women do, in fact, differ from one another: some incorporate a maternal, nurturant manner, while others reject or suppress such behavior as nonsurgeonlike. Consequently, the surgeons may indicate with perfect truth that some women are abrupt with patients, while some men are compassionate. I will argue, however, that *men and women are compassionate in different ways: men are fatherly, not motherly.* (These issues are discussed in Chapter 6.)

Concepts of embodied identity mediate between theories which assume that women are essentially different from men and those which define gender as an "interactional achievement" influenced solely by the situation. Unlike the theories of radical social constructionists, the notion of habitus does not take it for granted that humans are infinitely plastic, able to undergo rapid and revolutionary transformation as a response to altered social arrangements. The habitus molds individuals who embody the dominant modes of thought and experience in their social worlds (see Robbins 1991: 84). Such embodiment is relatively inflexible: these individuals look, feel, behave like members of their particular gender, class, group. These members then transmit to the next generation the embodied values and behavior of their group or class.

Such inflexibility might well be interpreted as biology by an observer. Difference exists—true difference, deep difference. And although such internalized and embodied difference is socially transmitted and alters through time, it is relatively resistant to abstract programs of planned change.[43] These embodied aspects of the habitus appear natural to actors and observers when both are situated in the same invisible social matrix. Biological or genetic explanations are then offered to account for these "natural" differences.

Compared to the certainties of biological reductionism, or the dualities of the difference theorists, social constructionist explanations based on "doing" or "negotiating" gender are helpful in explaining a wide variety of observed behavior. The problems with such an approach, however, are highlighted by a recent attempt to describe race and class, as well as gender, as "ongoing interactional accomplishments" (West and Fenstermaker 1995). Social interaction may express difference; it may magnify, or even create difference; but difference is surely not limited to interaction. Race, class, and gender inhere in *bodies,* tangible bodies as well as "imaginary bodies"—those images, symbols, and beliefs that shape social and political reality for individuals and groups (Gatens 1996: viii).[44]

Yes, gender is a process that is "negotiated" and "done." Yes, it is affected by conflict over scarce resources and social relationships of power, where men as a group benefit from the subordination of women as a group (Lorber 1994). But why, then, do some women enthusiastically help sabotage other, more powerful women, while just as enthusiastically serving dominant men? Interpretations based almost solely on self-interest, blindness, or ignorance seem insufficient and patronizing. I turned to the idea of embodiment not to replace analyses of doing and negotiating gender or explanations based on scarce resources and power relationships, but to supplement these with a more flexible, sensitive, and powerful way of explaining difference.[45]

Steering between biological essentialism and utter social plasticity, we can employ the notion of embodied identity to illuminate the workings of the social construction of gender. We need neither reject difference when we find it, nor insist on finding it. What we must reject are ideologies which maintain that difference is innately deep—or negligibly shallow. Difference may be deep, and difficult to alter or eradicate, yet it may not be essential. Gender is done, negotiated, socially produced, but it is real, as real as any other social phenomenon that structures our experience, our bodies, our behavior, our values, and our lives.

I began my study by looking for difference. Observing the way patients, nurses, chiefs of surgery, colleagues, and residents imposed their own cultural categories of difference upon women surgeons, I started to explore the social construction of difference. Although I collected a rich body of data, the concepts of "doing" or "negotiating" gender seemed insufficient to explain what was occurring. I observed women surgeons learning, accepting, negotiating, and resisting "categories of difference." But this was not all that was going on. The women were not merely acted on, or even reacting. Gender was not just a theoretical category or interactional achievement. It was not simply something the women thought or even performed. Gender, I concluded, is deeper, less intellectualized, more powerful than such formulations suggest. "Learned by body" from day one, gender inheres in the woman; it is not merely imposed on her.

In some ways I have come full circle. Without adopting "essentialist" notions, this book will examine what I first started to investigate: differences between women surgeons and their male colleagues. The women do differ from the men. (Even those who behave like their male colleagues differ from them.) They must, for extrinsic and intrinsic reasons. Naturally, they differ from one another as well, and differ *in* their differences. In this book, I will attempt to explore not only differences—and similarities—but when and how such differences are displayed, and the internal and external forces that affect them.

# TELLING STORIES

In the early 1970s, when I was drafting my dissertation on the contemporary American women's movement, it did not occur to me to question my adviser's counsel to avoid writing in the first person. To my astonishment, Victor Turner, an anthropologist whose work I admired and revered, asked me to put myself back into the text before he considered it for publication. This would have required not only time and effort, but a kind of emotional clarity that I was not yet ready to risk. In order to insert myself into the story, I would have had to take a good hard look at myself, my life, my marriage, and the reasons I was interested in the feminist movement. I published the impersonal version. Had I possessed the courage and ability to present my own self and motives in relation to those of the women I investigated, the book would have been more interesting, more perceptive, and more profound.

Gradually, I've found my voice. No longer influenced by my professors, I am now convinced that the most effective way (for me, at least) to present findings based on individual observations is to represent myself as an emotionally engaged participant, interacting with the people I study (Tedlock 1991).[1] "Narrative ethnography" is more interesting to read, more satisfying to write.

Although Barbara Tedlock (1991: 85) lists a number of narrative accounts of anthropological research published since 1980 by both men and women, it is my impression that more have been produced by women.[2] This makes sense theoretically, culturally, and historically. There is a rough (and unspoken) division of anthropological labor: men write theory; women tell stories. Is this because women in Western culture are more accustomed to expressing themselves through storytelling? (My daughter, a linguist, contends that women tell stories to hold the wandering attention of men, who prefer to hear themselves talking.) Or is it because when male anthropologists tell stories, their writing, as Catherine Lutz puts it (1990: 621), self-consciously "presents itself, through various often-subtle devices, as 'cutting edge' or avant-garde"? Lutz points out not only that the styles and approaches associated with the male are more highly valued, but also that a particular approach or style, whether produced by a man or a woman, may be evaluated with as much reference to gender stereotypes as to the intrinsic qualities of the text. Thus, men's stories are extolled as experimental "dialogical" anthropology, while women's are ignored or perceived as uncomfortably subjective.[3]

Perhaps, as Tedlock asserts, anthropology is going through a "representational transformation," with narrative anthropology becoming an accepted, even preferred, mode of presenting the dialogue between self and other. But perhaps not.[4] Tedlock's argument ignores the scientism and "physics envy" that permeate the human sciences. Telling stories is too much fun, reading stories is too accessible, to be identified as true scholarship, which ideally should be cerebral, remote, analytic, and polysyllabic. Theory, in other words, must announce itself as such (Lutz 1995: 252–254); it cannot quietly sneak up on the reader without being perceived as "mere description."[5]

Nevertheless, I write the kind of ethnographies I most enjoy reading. On occasion, I use traditional social science mechanisms: citations, analyses, generalizations. Whenever possible, however, I prefer to present concepts in narrative form. Stories are one of the oldest, most elementary, most elemental forms of human communication; every culture possesses stories that impart values, concepts, behaviors.

Western medicine, too, relies on stories to teach and communicate (Hunter 1991), and many doctors are superlative storytellers. Lacking the gifts of poet or philosopher, I cannot create archetypal narratives. I can, however, use narrative to convey some of my findings. Here, then, is the story of a day spent with a woman surgeon.

## HEADACHE CAPITAL OF THE WORLD

At the end of office hours, Hannah Krieger, a breast surgeon at a university hospital, asked a Breast Service secretary if she had any painkiller. "Yes, I've got the good stuff—Motrin 600," the woman responded. "This is headache capital of the world!" Half-jokingly she asked me, "You want one too?"

It had been a long day, and there was more to come. I met Dr. Krieger at 7:30 A.M. at the office where she saw patients (she had another, for academic activities). She wore a nylon print dress with pleated skirt, black patent leather shoes with tiny heels, medium-sized diamond stud earrings, and a green glass necklace. "I try not to make a fashion statement," she said. The dress was covered by a white lab coat, pockets filled with gear, including a bulging loose-leaf notebook that went everywhere with her. I was not surprised to see a framed certificate on her consulting room wall from Alpha Omega Alpha, the medical honor society.

In my fieldnotes, I observed: "I have loads of fieldnotes. Partly because Krieger says so much so fast; and much of it is so interesting and funny, and some so intelligent and compassionate, that I keep trying to write it down. Her staccato delivery is a particular New York phenomenon that I had forgotten. I hear my own New York accent emerging as I converse with her!"

We began at 8:00 A.M. with a meeting of the Ethics Committee. Krieger told me she made time for this because some of the best minds at the hospital were members and she found their discussions stimulating. So did I. There was none of the competitive intellectual display that I've observed at other such gatherings; instead, the members focused entirely on the problems at hand. The discussion was brilliant, fascinating, and enlightening. Although various abstract issues were touched on, the focus was on finding the most effective course of action in each case presented. Afterward, Krieger told me that she particularly liked and respected the committee's chair, a pulmonary specialist in his sixties: "I want to be like him when I grow up!" declared the thirty-seven-year-old surgeon. Later, she made the same statement about a pediatric surgeon who had gone out of his way to call her about a neighbor's child he had just operated on. "He didn't *have* to call me," she said. "He's got everything: clinical skill, moral integrity—he's a wonderful surgeon. I want to be like him when I grow up!"

On the way back to her office, Krieger told me that she was having a barbecue that weekend for everyone in the Breast Service: doctors, secretaries, nurses, technicians. It seemed amazing that a woman who had two young children, and who spent a couple of hours each day on the subway commuting to an arduous job, could manage to fit entertaining into her schedule, but I had already learned that being a woman surgeon, especially a married woman with children, was a high-metabolism pursuit. Krieger declared that she was taking the following Monday off; I assumed she wished to clean up and recuperate from the barbecue. As emergencies erupted during the day, however, and patients whose biopsies showed malignancies needed to see her to discuss the alternatives, Krieger kept offering to come in early Monday morning to discuss it with them. One woman took her up on the offer. I observed in my fieldnotes: "To be a compassionate surgeon, especially . . . with breasts, means not worrying about one's time but giving everything the time it needs, no matter how much time that is . . . Pamela Pearson [a well-known breast surgeon in another city whom I had observed at work] doesn't do this [discuss the alternatives at length with worried patients]; her nurse does. I keep looking at the breast surgeons, thinking: Who would I use if I had a malignant lump?"

After the Ethics Committee meeting, Krieger had office hours. She saw nine patients, spending a great deal of time with each, giving careful explanations in simple language, explaining what might happen, what the percentages were, what choices were available, how the patient would feel after a procedure, and how the patient's breast would look. Frequently, the husbands were present. Krieger said she encourages husbands to participate; she tries to give them emotional support, she said, so that they can support their wives. I noticed that unlike most surgeons I've observed, she did not use the term "incision"—she just pointed. I always wondered whether patients understood the word. No visit was terminated until Krieger had answered every question that the patient and her husband had. Several times, a worried patient asked the same question over and over in different words; each time, Krieger responded, showing no sign of impatience. When a woman clasped her hands or hugged her, Krieger clasped or hugged back; she was clearly comfortable with body contact, and her demeanor indicated that she was physically and emotionally approachable.

She said she had worked until 8:00 P.M. the previous day.

"What did you do about dinner?" I asked, and she replied that she had tried to eat it when she got home, at 9:00 P.M. During the day, she phoned her husband and talked with him; her tone was one of loving comradeship. She told me how her younger daughter had said she wanted a baby boy: "It's like wanting a dog—she wants a baby," said Krieger. "I told her that God doesn't always plan things like that, but she didn't hear me." I looked at the framed photos of two little girls in her consulting room and commented on the devilish look in the little one's eyes. "Yes, she's impish," said Krieger, "and the big one is so sweet. They're really wonderful girls!"

There was a pause between patients, and Krieger made some phone calls. She began with the negative biopsies, the ones that showed no malignancy. "Now we've got the tough ones coming up," she murmured, "so let's start with the least hard of the bad ones." She was obviously talking to herself. "Hi, Mrs. Barish, it's Dr. Krieger. How are you? We got the reports back. There was some breast cancer. It extended into the skin, that's why it looked like that. It was shallow and extended, rather than deep. I want to talk to you. You and your husband are coming into the office and we're going to talk. You've got some options and decisions." The patient asked a question. "I have no reason to believe this is an advanced cancer of any sort. This is *not* an advanced cancer and you had a negative mammogram and we felt nothing in the nodes, so it's probably not at all advanced. Come in late this afternoon," Krieger suggested. "What time? Before 2:00, if possible. How late is 'later than 2:00'? If you can come in at 2:30, okay." When she hung up, Krieger said to me, "She's older—that's always a little easier. This other one we're going to tell [of a positive biopsy] is going to flip major league."

She told me that one old lady was coming to see her from a nursing home. The woman had been a high school French teacher, and she "recursed," saying over and over, "Vous êtes une bonne femme. Je vous aime." "She's adorable," said Krieger. The patient was in the waiting area with a nursing-home attendant, but Krieger was waiting for the woman's granddaughter before seeing the old lady. When the granddaughter arrived, she came into the secretaries' office to talk with Krieger. The women hugged each other. The young woman was worried: her grandmother appeared to be failing. The granddaughter's eyes and nose turned red, and she began to cry. Krieger left the office, returning with a tiny box of Kleenex which she handed to the young woman. "Look how long we've kept her going," said Krieger, reminding her that her grandmother had been diagnosed with Stage 3 cancer three years before (a Stage 3 cancer is very advanced but not metastatic).

Next on the schedule was a biopsy, performed in a little "procedure room" in the Breast Service suite. There were five women in the room: the patient, the doctor, a nurse, a "physician's assistant," and me, the anthropologist-observer. The patient appeared to be in her late sixties or early seventies. "Doctor, I want you to examine me—all my breasts," said the patient. "*All* your breasts!" said Krieger in a teasing tone. She examined the woman and reassured her that there were no new findings. After scrubbing, and donning a gown and gloves, Krieger inquired about the cassette player that the physician's assistant sometimes brought to work: "You didn't bring it? Okay, I won't sing." The patient told Krieger she could sing if she wanted to. "Trust me on this one," responded Krieger. "You don't want me to. I'm terrifically enthusiastic, but not very talented." She said to the nurse, "Although we have sung for patients, haven't we?" As she talked in a reassuring tone, she was working. "I'm going to tell you when you'll feel a little stick. A little stick," she said, injecting lidocaine into the biopsy site, "then some burning. If you count to ten, you won't feel anything by the time you get to ten. You'll know something is going on but you won't feel anything." She announced, "I'm just about done. The lump is tiny." When the patient expressed surprise that it was so fast, the surgeon said, making a gesture indicating that she was joking: "We were thinking of doing a long operation with lots of complicated stuff. I was definitely considering that!" The patient kept quizzing her about what she found. "What I see?" responded Krieger. I don't see anything suspicious. It's very very small. This will have to be a microscopic diagnosis." The patient kept questioning: If it was bad, would she need radiation? When would Krieger call her? Krieger gave reassuring but utterly truthful responses. "What do you see? What do you think?" the patient kept asking. "I don't *see* anything suspicious, but I don't know. You can't push me any further. I just don't know," Krieger declared.

On the way back from the procedure room, we passed the waiting area. The old lady from the nursing home was making a terrific ruckus, talking and singing at the top of her lungs. "Put her in the examining room, she's clearing the waiting room," Krieger directed. Before seeing her, Krieger told me that the patient was ninety-seven and would soon be ninety-eight. She had an advanced breast tumor, but was too old and had too many diseases to be operated on; the diseases or old age might well kill her before the cancer did. The granddaughter was very devoted. She had been the one to find Krieger, and she brought her grandmother in from a suburban nursing home. It was a wonderful family, Krieger declared, and the attendant who was accompanying the woman was very good too.

Into the examining room we went, where the patient was already installed. The old lady was completely out of it. She insisted on eating her third sandwich, and refused to be examined. "I see you've got a new haircut," Krieger said to her. "Punk. I like it, it's really cool." The patient's thinning hair stood up in frizzy coils. "Isn't it great!" the granddaughter chorused. The old lady refused to be examined and demanded another sandwich. Krieger was warm and patient. "Give her the other sandwich, we'll try after that," she directed. "I'll make a bargain with you," she said coaxingly to the patient, but the old lady was not listening. She spoke French, sang in a rather attractive operatic voice, yelled, and chanted. The granddaughter, Krieger, and the male attendant all tried to coax her to allow her breast to be examined. Ignoring them, the patient bit into her sandwich. "Peanut butter, I love peanut butter," said Krieger, but the old lady tore the sandwich to pieces and decided she didn't want it. "Skin like silk!" said the attendant in a cajoling tone. "That's what she says," confided the granddaughter, and indeed the old lady's facial skin was very soft. "Why don't you show it to the doctor," continued the attendant. "You don't like me," said the patient sulkily to the attendant. "You like those fat old women!" "Oh no," chorused Krieger and the granddaughter. "How could he like a fat old woman when he's got a cute little one like you!" Finally the old lady allowed her undershirt to be lifted and her breast examined. The breast looked raw, with terrible-looking lesions on and under it. "We're holding our own," said Krieger. It didn't look this way to the worried granddaughter. "She *is* loonier," agreed Krieger, saying that this was not due to the cancer; if it were, the patient would show neurological deficits. "It's just that all systems are going," she explained.

Krieger told the granddaughter that they could not operate: the patient would probably die on the table. She did, however, use the examining-room telephone to consult a medications expert about the tranquilizer the old lady was taking; learning that a stronger dose was safe, she wrote a prescription and gave it to the granddaughter. She also wrote a message on the chart for the nursing home, informing them that the drug increased appetite and advising them to give the old lady all the food she wanted. The granddaughter thanked her, saying that her grandmother was difficult. "Oh no, she's adorable!" said Krieger, who had again been told in French that she was a very good woman whom the patient loved. "That's you!" said the granddaughter. "Lots of people have trouble with her."

The next patient was Mrs. Barish, whom Krieger had telephoned about the biopsy and whom she had squeezed into that day's office hours. The patient looked like my Aunt Mary, complete with the leathery skin of a sun-worshiper. Krieger went through the choices: There were two alternatives. The first one had three parts. If the patient chose it, she had to go through all three parts—lumpectomy, node dissection, radiation. The second alternative was mastectomy. Nodes would be removed at the same time the breast was removed, and no radiation would be necessary. Krieger's description of the choices was a model of clarity and simplicity—the sort that's more difficult to achieve than complexity.[6] Later, when I complimented her on it, she responded that she had spent a long time figuring out "that spiel," to make it understandable to patients. There were many questions from Mrs. and Mr. Barish, including a long recital, which Krieger had obviously heard before, about Mrs. Barish's previous bouts with cancer. Together, Krieger and the Barishes discussed how best to schedule the procedure to coincide with a planned trip to Israel. When leaving, Mrs. Barish said: "I don't know why this happened. As I told you, my father was an Orthodox rabbi. Someone up there mustn't like me!" "I don't know the answer to that," responded Krieger in a gentle tone, "and if I did, I wouldn't be doing this—I'd be in the stock market!"

"Now I'll take a Valium and make the worst phone call," said Krieger. The patient was not home. Krieger talked to the woman's husband, carefully answering every question, although she knew she'd have to go through the same questions with the patient. "She's going to have to have more surgery. This is her worst nightmare!" Krieger said. She told the husband not to give the patient the news—just to tell her to call the doctor. "Your wife needs to look at you as her comfort and support, not the messenger of bad news," she said, adding, "You have been superb! The two of you will get through this. She will get through this. She won't have to like it—she won't enjoy anything about it. But she will get through this." She kept repeating the phrase with great conviction and emphasis. She pointed out to the husband that the patient's mother had been diagnosed with a very bad disease, but that the patient herself had *not* been diagnosed with a bad disease. Later, Krieger told me that the patient's mother had "died like a dog" of breast cancer, and her aunt as well, so the patient had "lost it" when she'd had to have a biopsy. She'd become so hysterical that they'd had to sedate her and put her in a wheelchair to get her to the operating room. After Krieger hung up, she said to me, "You can see why I go home every night with a headache!" When I said that I understood, and that she still had to talk to the patient, she responded, "Yes. But it's very good work. It's very good work," she repeated with conviction. "It's important and it's necessary, and everyone in this office believes that, from the file clerk on up. It's very good work."

The next patient was a twenty-eight-year-old woman who gave an excruciatingly precise history. She had come for a second opinion: her breast surgeon had found nothing and had told her there was nothing wrong, but she was convinced she felt something and that it was getting larger. When asked about past illnesses, she related how one doctor had said she might have a prolapsed heart valve; this was disproved, but she was continuing to take antibiotics whenever she went to the dentist, just in case. When questioned about allergies, she said she was allergic to smoked salmon and Neutrogena soap, but not to shellfish. Asked about drugs, she carefully said that her ear-nose-and-throat doctor had prescribed special nose-drops, but that she had not yet filled the prescription. When we had first entered the waiting room to fetch her, Krieger had pointed to me in my white lab coat, and had asked the patient if it was okay if Dr. Cassell sat in, adding that I was spending the day observing. The patient had assented. Now, before leaving the consulting room to enter the examining room, Krieger asked again if it was okay if I observed, and again the patient assented. Krieger examined the woman's breasts. "I can't find anything. Is it here?" she inquired, feeling the right breast. No, it was not there, said the patient. "Get dressed and we'll talk," said Krieger. While waiting for the patient to join us in the consulting room, Krieger said, "I always tell patients to get dressed. Nobody should have to talk with their clothes off." The patient entered. Krieger told her that she had found nothing significant, that the patient just had "nodular breasts." The patient asked question after question: Why had Krieger asked if she was allergic to shellfish? What had she felt when she asked, 'Is it here?' What did 'nodular breasts' mean? Endless and sometimes repetitive questions, all of which Krieger answered with no sign of impatience. When the patient left, Krieger told me she was a lawyer. I remembered my former husband, an internist, telling me that female lawyers are horrendous patients.

Krieger then got a call from the patient who was sure to be upset by her positive biopsy. "This is an early breast cancer," Krieger said. "This is not advanced. This is not neglected. This is early breast cancer, and in 1994 we have a lot of options open to you. Yeah, I know it's a shock." Krieger kept talking and talking; it was obvious that the patient was hysterical and not hearing very much she was saying. Later, Krieger told me that the patient had said the best thing she could do was to jump off the Triboro Bridge. During this phone conversation, Krieger was buzzed three times. The second two times, after asking the patient to hold, she said in an impatient tone: "Yes!" Once it was the woman in charge of billing: the lawyer was making a fuss about the bill. Krieger told the woman not to buzz her, she was occupied and did not want to discuss it with the patient, who was demanding to talk to her. She went back to the hysterical patient on the telephone, saying: "We have a complete team involved—radiologists, a psychiatrist, mammographers, nurses, breast surgeons, all at your behest. You have the advantage of early diagnosis, and that's a big advantage. It's very very treatable. In 1994, it is one of the most treatable diseases. If you choose to seek an opinion elsewhere, that's fine. It can help make you more confident about our decision." She must have been on the phone for fifteen or twenty minutes, and finally arranged to see the patient first thing Monday morning. In my fieldnotes, I observed: "Bet it takes two or three hours, on what's supposed to be her day off."

After Krieger hung up, her secretary called. The lawyer was "tearing up the place." She was enraged at the $250 fee for a second opinion. "I don't want to talk to her. We'll wait here till she's left," said Krieger. But when she got a second call from the woman in billing, telling her that the patient had said she was "humiliated" at having "an intern" there watching, and that she was telling everyone, including patients in the waiting area, how badly she'd been treated, Krieger said, "Send her in." Krieger was trembling with anger. (She later told me that she'd had a terrible temper as a child, and that she had made a great effort to control it and had succeeded; but that when she *did* get angry she got *really* angry.) "Come in," she said icily to the patient. "Did you say you were humiliated that Dr. Cassell was there?" she inquired. "Didn't you agree twice to have her observe?" "That isn't what I said—your employee lied," responded the patient. "Listen to what I said. Listen to what I have to say. Listen." "Okay, I'll listen to what you have to say," responded Krieger.

The patient then declared that she had said she was "insulted" not "humiliated," that she had said yes to being observed just in order to be "a good egg," but that $250 was outrageous. Her breast surgeon charged only $50, and he was a Fifth Avenue doctor; and her dermatologist charged $85. She paid $250 when she went to her internist for a complete physical, with tests and everything. Besides, Krieger hadn't even looked at the mammogram; she had spent only ten or fifteen minutes with her, and so far as she could tell, Krieger hadn't even looked at the mammogram. The woman stopped, with an air of triumph, as though she had just voiced an irrefutable argument. "Have you said what you have to say?" inquired Krieger. The patient assented.

Krieger then told her that $250 was the office fee for a second opinion, that this fee was not just for her but for every patient. She said that the patient had agreed twice to allow Dr. Cassell to observe, and that Dr. Cassell had not touched her or interfered in any way. And as for mammograms, the "standard of care" was to have a mammographer read them, and the patient's had been read by Dr. Carey, the head of the Breast Service mammography unit. The radiologist had found nothing significant—here it was on her chart. The patient attempted to speak, but Krieger cut her off. "It's my turn to speak now," she declared, telling the woman that she was not going to discuss fees with her. "That's not my job—that's why we have someone in billing to discuss money," she said. "But if you think the fee is unfair, here's what I'm going to do." She tore the bill into several pieces and said, "That's it! You pay nothing. There's no fee for your consultation!" The patient tried to say that she was willing to pay something "fair," $70 or even $125, but Krieger would not listen. "I don't argue about money. There's no fee," she declared. The patient hesitated by her desk, as though she wanted to say something. Krieger buzzed her secretary and said, "Ms. Kafavy is coming to get her chart. She can get her mammograms downstairs," making it clear that the interview was terminated. She was trembling with rage. "I'm going to think about this all weekend. One more fucking deadbeat!" she said. She told me that the previous Christmas her partner had purchased an inflatable reproduction of the figure depicted in Edvard Munch's painting *The Scream* and had installed it in the office. "We loved it," she said. "That's how I feel much of the time." They had finally decided that it wasn't appropriate for patients to see the figure, and they'd put it away; but she'd really loved having it there.

It was 4:00 P.M. Office hours were finally over. Krieger had seen nine women, including two on whom she had performed biopsies. She made another phone call, to a patient with newly diagnosed cancer, but no one was home. She left a message and decided to make rounds. She said she had two mastectomy patients in the hospital: one was a bit "thick"; the other was "difficult."

The first stop was the "Tower," a luxurious high-rise facility for patients. Mrs. Fleisher had undergone a mastectomy the previous day. Krieger had described the procedure to me. The patient was a three-hundred-pound woman whose breasts came down, literally, to her knees. It had taken three hours to do the mastectomy. At the same time, the plastic surgeon had reduced the size of the second breast. When Krieger, a small woman, had tried to carry the tissue from both breasts to the refrigerator (where it was to be held for analysis), the breast tissue had been too heavy for her to budge. Mrs. Fleisher turned out to be an Orthodox Jew wearing a turban; her husband had a beard and wore a yarmulke. On the bedside table was an electric candle with two illuminated lights (it was Friday afternoon, and the Jewish Sabbath would soon begin). The patient had a broad peasant face; she spoke almost no English, just Spanish and Hebrew. Krieger talked to her in Spanish (which she had picked up during her residency) and English. The patient and her husband did not know how to straighten the hospital bed from its flexed position, and she had not left the bed since the operation. Krieger told her firmly that she had to move or she would get sick; she told the husband the same thing, but it was unclear how much they understood. It was more than linguistic incomprehension. Krieger had described them as "simple" people; she must have intended the term in the old-fashioned sense of "intellectually slow." She told me that the couple were South Americans who lived in an Orthodox Jewish enclave in Brooklyn. A few members of their community came to her as patients, and they sent others. The couple had little money, but in the expensive hotel-like Tower, the husband could stay overnight and order kosher meals for both of them. When we left, I said "Gut Shabbas" (which I remember my father saying), and Krieger said "Shabat Shalom." ("Gut Shabbas" is a Yiddish phrase meaning "Have a good Sabbath." "Shabat Shalom" is a Hebrew response wishing the other a peaceful and happy Sabbath.) Krieger then went to find the nurse to make sure the patient was helped, indeed forced, to walk. "There she is, three hundred pounds, lying there like a beached whale. That woman is a pulmonary embolism waiting to happen!"

We then visited an old lady who did nothing but complain. She began the moment Krieger entered the room: this hurts and that hurts, and this stings, and she coughs and coughs. "Why don't you take your pain medications?" demanded Krieger, but the patient was too busy complaining to respond. Krieger told her that she needed to cough because her lungs were filled with fluid from being anesthetized, and that she should hug a pillow to her when she coughed, so it would hurt less. The patient kept complaining about the cough, disregarding the doctor's advice. The complaints had a frantic, obsessive quality. The patient was in her seventies, and lived alone but had an unmarried son living nearby. "He's a pocket-protector kind of guy," said Krieger. "He wears pocket protectors, and he's got tape on the temple piece of his eyeglasses. Know what I mean?" I knew what she meant. I said I thought the old lady was a bit demented. "At first I thought she was just a cranky old lady," responded Krieger, "but it's more."

We visited one more patient: Krieger's secretary at another hospital, where she practices one day a week. It was a pleasure to listen to an intelligent, upbeat patient, although, as Krieger pointed out afterward, this woman was probably sicker than the previous two—suffering from metastatic disease and muscular degeneration (caused by early polio).

Krieger led me to the hospital's main entrance and indicated the route to the subway. As we walked, she discussed the barbecue scheduled for the coming weekend. I inquired about the menu. "I told you I'm a very good cook, and I love barbecues," she declared, itemizing the sumptuous menu.

She planned to go across the street to the children's hospital, to visit a neighbor's child who had just been operated on; then to her academic office in another part of the hospital, where she had left the jacket she'd been wearing when she arrived; and then home. I left her at 5:10. I had heard her tell her husband, on the telephone, that she would be home at 5:00. I thought to myself that she would be lucky if she arrived there at 6:30. Especially since I'd heard someone accost her after we parted: "Dr. Krieger!" It was probably a patient or family member requesting information and reassurance. I was exhausted. It was all I could do to get home, consume a take-out supper, and collapse. And I did not have a husband, two young children, and barbecue preparations waiting.

## RESURRECTING LAZARUS

Dr. Krieger specialized in breast surgery. Her partner, chief of the Breast Service, was also a woman, as were the three radiologists, who performed only mammograms. On occasion, I've wondered whether breast surgery might not be becoming a women's subspecialty. (As with women's studies, I've also wondered whether or not this was a good thing.)

Why do so many women enter this relatively low-prestige surgical specialty? Because they find the problems challenging? Because they want to help other women? When I interviewed Dr. Krieger about her surgical training and her thoughts on the differences between men and women surgeons, she related a story that illuminated some of the reasons women might choose this subspecialty. In a tape-recorded interview, I asked how she had coped with the rigors of surgical training.[7]

> *Dr. Krieger:* Toward the end of my chief residency I stopped coping . . . After so many years I just started to understand that no matter what I did, it wasn't going to work. I was never going to be equal, and I was never going to be looked at equally. There was one particular incident that sort of set this thing off . . . I think one of the reasons I had such a hard time is because I really thought, *I truly believed* for a number of years, that if I just worked hard and did right that I would be equal. That there was no way I would be denied. That I would just—I would just

prove that I was as good as anybody else and they would *have* to believe that. And that was proved to be a lie.

*Anthropologist:* What was the incident?

*Dr. Krieger:* [It] happened in the spring of my chief residency . . . I was chief resident at the VA [Veterans' Administration Hospital], and the chief residents in the VA took calls from home. And I was covering one weekend, and the second-year resident called me at home . . . in the middle of the afternoon on Saturday to say, panicked—this was a not very talented second-year resident—panicked, because he said to me, "There's a guy in the emergency room and he's eviscerated." I said, "Okay, who operated on him?" I figured he'd dehisced his wound post-op. He said, "He wasn't operated on, but he's eviscerated." I said, "Okay, Chuck, calm down, I'll be right there." Because clearly I'm not going to get any information from this guy over the phone . . . I put my shoes on and I walked over. And sure enough, there was this poor old vet in the emergency room with his small bowel all over his belly. And what basically had happened is, this was a guy with very, very bad cirrhosis of the liver who had very bad ascites. And he had had an umbilical hernia, and this is something that is recognized happens occasionally. He popped his hernia at home, and his guts came out and it sort of sat there for a couple of days. And he came out of his alcoholic stupor long enough to show up at the VA. It also turns out that he had an extensive medical history—had had coronary artery bypass surgery, median sternotomy—and now he's eviscerated. So we got the guy organized—clearly he was going to need to go to the operating room—got him moved up to the ICU, and we're getting ready to prepare to take him to the operating room. I asked the second-year resident to do some appropriate things, including putting in a Swan Ganz catheter, and a Foley, and all kinds of other jazz. And I went off to start to marshal the forces to come in. At the VA, this is a big deal. Nobody's there. We had to open the operating room on a Saturday. In the VA, you needed an act of Congress to do this! So I called up the nursing staff and I called anesthesia and I called the attending who was covering me at the time, and I said, "There's a guy, I think he's popped an umbilical hernia," and I gave him the whole story. So the attending said to me, "Okay, fix it." I said, "Do you have any other advice?" [laughter] "No, no, just fix it." I said, "Well, I figured that out already, thank you very much." And I hung up the phone. The second-year resident was having a tough time putting the Swan Ganz in because the guy had had a median sternotomy, and also he was *very* dehydrated at this point. So I went there . . . and I got the line in. While we're waiting for the OR to be opened, we get a chest X-ray. He has a small pneumothorax from the line insertion. Okay, that's okay, it happens. We put a chest tube in. He's perfectly fine. We go to the operating room. The second-year resident falls asleep; I have to throw him out of the OR. I open the abdomen. He has liters and liters and liters of ascites and terrible cirrhosis. I drain the ascites, I resect the small bowel, I put it back together. I debride the abdominal wall, which is all necrotic from all this stuff hangin' out, close him real tight and take him to the ICU. And lo and behold, ten days later the guy's off my service: he's on the rehab service, perfectly healed!

*Anthropologist:* It's a miracle.

*Dr. Krieger:* A miracle. And it's an interesting case. And it went well. I presented the case at an M & M conference that we had, and I thought, "This is a great case."

*Anthropologist:* It's really pretty cool, yes.

*Dr. Krieger:* This is pretty impressive—this is a great case! But the chairman was not there that day, and the rounds were being run by the next most senior attending . . . And . . . I presented this history. So the first thing they did, they spent fifteen minutes torturing me over this pneumothorax: "What had happened?" "What was the lighting?" "What was the this?" "What was the that?" The guy was dehydrated and had had a median sternotomy and he got a pneumothorax. And I took full responsibility—never mentioned the other resident involved. But, you know, I just didn't get it—I didn't get why this was such a big deal. Then we moved on. Then they wanted to talk about the performance of the surgery, and one of the senior attendings raised his hand and said, Why didn't I bring out the stomas? Why did I put it back together again? Why didn't I bring the ends out? I said, well, the patient had massive ascites—that's a relative contraindication to the formation of stomas. Plus the fact this was proximal small bowel; there was no reason not to make it an anastomosis in this setting. It wasn't pus in the abdomen—it was just ascites. And I basically justified myself medically. And his response was, "Well, *if* it had been just a little small bowel, *if* there was massive ascites, you should have brought the ends out." I'm like, "Yeah, well, so big deal." So that was another ten minutes. Now the last thing is, the senior attending who's running rounds says to me—I'm still standing up there, I've been there twenty minutes now, and this is not going well, I'm sensing that this is not going well—he says to me, "Well, after you closed the abdomen, did you leave the skin open?" And I said, "Well, we debrided the abdominal wall. We closed the abdomen and left the skin open." He said, "Did he leak ascites through his closure?" I said, "No." He said, "Wait a minute—he didn't leak at all?" I said, "No, he didn't," which was the absolute truth. He said, "Well, the last patient that I closed with massive ascites leaked terribly through the wound." I said, "Well, this patient didn't leak." So he concluded the discussion by saying, "Well, I guess I'd rather be lucky than smart."

*Anthropologist:* That son-of-a-bitch!

*Dr. Krieger:* And then I knew. And then I had that flash. And I said—the way I commented on this afterwards when I reported this incident to everybody who would stand still long enough to hear the story—I said, "If I reported at M & M that I had resurrected Lazarus, they would ask me why I'd waited four days!"

She added that the next presentation at the M & M conference had been by another chief resident, "one of the chosen few," who had described a relatively simple case: a patient had bled after having his thyroid removed and, because of respiratory difficulties, the incision had had to be opened at the bedside. In contrast to the fault-finding that greeted her spectacular "save," this young man "was held as a hero of modern medicine."[8] "So that just did it," Krieger concluded. "That just cut it. That was the end. That was the end."

Dr. Krieger's story sounded familiar. But I did not realize *how* familiar until I began to write this chapter. To repeat Catherine Lutz's insight from her discussion of the "erasure of women's voices": not only are the styles and approaches associated with men more highly valued than those of women, but a particular approach or style, whether of a man or a woman, may be evaluated with as much reference to gender stereotypes as to its intrinsic qualities (1990: 621). To translate from anthropological to surgical terms, not only are dramatic macho "saves" valorized over compassionate, empathetic, clinically informed surgical care, but when women *do* perform dramatic saves, the male audience assumes that something inevitably must have been done wrong.

Hannah Krieger learned, during her training, that (to paraphrase her words) no matter what she did, it wasn't going to work. She was never going to be equal, and she was never going to be looked at equally. After spending a year conducting research, and two and a half years practicing general surgery at a university hospital department of surgery which was undergoing political difficulties and upheavals, she accepted a position in the Breast Service of another university hospital. In the martial, male-identified world of surgery, breast surgery is one of the few subspecialties where being a woman is an advantage. Many women prefer to consult other women about their breasts. Even the most insensitive woman surgeon is unlikely to make the classic remark that several patients said they'd heard from men who were urging them to undergo an immediate mastectomy: "At your age, what do you need your breast for?"

In addition, many men prefer not to take on breast cases. Technically, the procedures (biopsies, node dissections, lumpectomies, mastectomies) are less challenging than the operations that general surgeons and oncologists (cancer specialists) delight in. In the early 1980s, a competent, compassionate, highly respected male surgeon performing a mastectomy said to me, "I hate this!" "Oh yes, it's so fraught!" I responded, thinking how crazed I would be at the prospect of losing a breast. "No, it's *boring!*" he responded. A breast surgeon rarely gets the opportunity to perform a dramatic save. At the same time, patients are frantic and terrified. A woman's breasts have enormous symbolic and psychic valence, and the prospect of losing one is paralyzing.[9]

A woman who had left general surgery to specialize in breast surgery told me that her colleagues regarded her with disdain: "I'm not a real surgeon any more." She described how a woman friend of hers, a general surgeon, had discouraged her from pursuing this subspecialty: "What, are you crazy?" the friend had exclaimed. After having a baby at the age of forty-one, however, the friend had indeed decided to concentrate on breasts. The schedules of breast surgeons are fairly manageable: middle-of-the night emergencies are exceptional, and the answering service can screen off-hour calls from distraught patients, if the surgeon so wishes.

Whether or not a woman surgeon is sensitive, compassionate, and caring, she is expected to be so, and such behavior is frequently elicited by patients, nurses, families, and even male colleagues, who may send women breast cases because they find them technically boring, because they prefer to avoid the emotional demands, or because they genuinely believe women will meet these demands more effectively. Naturally, women surgeons may differ from men not only in empathy and compassion, but also in the amount of time they are willing to spend in the office and on the telephone, listening to frantic women recurse—repeat the same question over and over.

Of the thirty-three women surgeons I studied, ten had a large number of breast patients. Of these, six identified themselves as breast specialists. Three were exceptionally empathetic and compassionate, spending hours in their offices and on the telephone, counseling and reassuring women so panicked that they were unable to hear what the surgeon was saying.[10] Of the three, Dr. Krieger stood out, not only for the clarity of her explanations and the extent of her patience, but also for the intensity and magnitude of her patients' demands. Some of this demanding behavior may have been due to her forbearance: she permitted patients to devour time—to talk, weep, have hysterics, telephone late at night and on weekends—whereas other surgeons I observed made it clear immediately that such behavior would not be tolerated. Some may have been due to the kind of patient who seeks or is sent to a university hospital specialist. For example, Ms. Kafavy, the lawyer who made a scene about her fee, had already consulted her internist and a breast surgeon before coming to Dr. Krieger; unable to allay her fears (and perhaps exhausted by her demands), the internist had "turfed" her to a breast surgeon, who had "turfed" her to the university hospital specialist. ("Turfing" a patient—usually one whose case or personality is difficult—involves referring him or her to another physician.) And some may have been due to inexperience: younger doctors, and Dr. Krieger had at that time been in practice only six years, permit behavior that more experienced doctors have learned to forestall or to turf.

One day, I was with Krieger when she received a phone call about a patient, whose case she subsequently described. An Italian woman in her forties, a professor of art history, had discovered a lump in her breast. She was in the midst of a divorce—her husband had left her for a younger woman. After the patient's biopsy revealed a malignancy, she insisted that her husband be at the hospital during the lumpectomy. She wanted Krieger to remove both breasts. Krieger refused; the tumor was small. She thought the patient wished to commit suicide in front of her husband, using Krieger as the means. Now, said Krieger, the woman had a recurrence of the cancer. The patient was taking bootleg (nonprescribed) estrogen obtained from a friend in Europe. Insisting she needed it to clear her mind and think properly, she refused to stop, despite the recurrence. (A number of studies indicate that estrogens may increase the severity of breast cancers.) Krieger went along with her at first, hoping to maintain the connection and work with the patient to convince her to take proper care of her disease. But not only was the woman taking bootleg Premarin; she was also manipulating her own medications. Krieger wanted her to begin taking an estrogen-blocking drug, which some studies had shown to be effective against breast cancer. But the woman insisted on being sent to one gynecologist after another, hoping to find someone who would prescribe estrogens. She wanted to continue the estrogen and also have a prophylactic mastectomy on the second breast. (Prophylactic mastectomies, which involve the removal of a breast that is not cancerous, are sometimes performed on patients who are at high risk of contracting breast cancer.)

During the woman's last office visit, when Krieger informed her that she had to take proper care of the first breast before Krieger would do anything about the second, the patient had ended up screaming at her. Krieger was now worried: going along with the patient's wishes would make *her* legally liable, since what the patient wanted, Premarin, was not what was best for her, nor was it the accepted course of surgical care. I told Krieger what I had learned as a doctor's wife: young doctors get the impossible patients—that's how they learn what they can and cannot do, and whom they can and cannot care for. Eventually, they know enough to send patients they cannot work with to other, younger doctors. "I can't sleep over this woman!" Krieger declared.

I suspect that every woman is as fear-haunted as I at the possibility of contracting breast cancer, and that, like me, every woman knows she may well be crazed with terror if a malignancy is found. Each time I observed a woman surgeon talk to a breast cancer patient, I wondered whether this was the surgeon I would choose if I contracted the disease. Of the three most compassionate surgeons I encountered, only one, Dr. Krieger, was at a first-rate hospital, with good nursing care and top-notch facilities. After studying her, I concluded that Krieger was the surgeon I would want: she was brilliant, careful, caring, knowledgeable, and well-trained.

Dr. Krieger was the breast surgeon many women might wish for. But she paid a price. Krieger had the true surgical temperament (Cassell 1991: 33–59). She loved to operate, and relished challenging cases and dramatic saves. When asked how she had become a surgeon, she said that she had wanted to be a pediatrician when she went to medical school, but in her third year, when she'd done a pediatric "rotation,"[11] she'd hated the fact that the children were always crying and that everything she did hurt them. She had then done a clerkship in surgery, mostly to get it out of the way:

> The interesting thing about it was that I *really* enjoyed it. I just had a terrific time. And I'm not just saying that I learned a lot, [that] it was challenging—I had *fun*, F-U-N. I mean this was fun. We did fun stuff! And I liked the immediacy of the patient's problem. I liked the idea of intervening directly and making a real difference, and not watching and waiting around . . . [She had then considered going into internal medicine] And I ultimately decided to do what I subjectively had liked better and where I had more *fun*. That's what it really came down to. This is what I *liked*.

Is breast surgery—with its comparatively simple technical requirements and enormously demanding patients—fun? Krieger was doing good work, necessary work, and knew it. But was she still having a lot of fun with it?

Dr. Krieger gave her distraught, demanding patients the sympathy and empathy they asked for. But day after day she went home with a headache, losing sleep over difficult patients. Would she have been as compassionate and empathetic a surgeon if she had avoided getting so close to patients, if she hadn't allowed herself to get so deeply involved? Perhaps older, more experienced breast surgeons have learned to tread a fine line between headache and empathy, between sleeplessness and involvement. On the other hand, perhaps only relatively young surgeons have the emotional energy to move in as close as she did—to listen to, hug, hold, and comfort patients as well as giving first-rate surgical care. If this is true, there may be certain advantages to choosing a young surgeon. Hysterics and "crazies" are not the only ones who need to be treated with patience, consideration, and compassion. Cancer is a terrible disease that is not so much cured as halted or arrested. And though a cure may be impossible, the surgeon can at least listen, bear witness, care *about* as well as *for* the patient. This is healing, not cure—part of the art, as opposed to the science, of surgery. Men as well as women practice this art: the former can be just as compassionate as the latter. Perhaps in the case of breast cancer, however, a *woman's* caring and empathy—when it is offered—has a more profound meaning to the patient. This leads to issues that will be explored in a later chapter: the difference between "maternal" and "paternal" bodies, behaviors, roles, relationships; the ways in which female and male surgeons relate to patients; and the ways in which patients relate to female and male surgeons.

# 4 / / / / / / / / / / / / / / / / / / / / /

# WOMEN LEADING

*First Vignette.* The patient was already under anesthesia when a young woman entered the OR and introduced herself to the surgeon, saying that she was a medical student. The celebrated surgeon, whom I'll call Dr. Adams, accompanied the student to the sink outside the OR, where they scrubbed together. The surgeon returned before the student, whose scrubbing seemed to take forever. "She very green, very green, so be nice to her, but watch her," the surgeon cautioned the scrub nurse. She told the assembled personnel that the patient was an ICU nurse in San Francisco who had "gone through networks" to get help after suffering from intractable pain for two years.

The surgeon began "opening" at 8:15 A.M. She was assisted by a chief resident and the student, and was observed by a visiting professor from Taiwan, who had told me that Dr. Adams was the best in the world in her particular subspecialty. He said he'd read her publications and felt privileged to watch her operate. A colleague entered and inquired about the case, which the surgeon described as she worked. "Margaret?" she inquired of the medical student. "Margareta," responded the student. "I'm going to keep saying it till I get it right," said the surgeon. A sizable group now circled the table: the medical student, the chief resident, a colleague who kept coming in to see what was going on, the scrub nurse, and the Taiwanese visitor.[1] As she worked, the surgeon described exactly what she was doing; she gave the rationale for each maneuver and quoted statistics from studies, some of which she had conducted.

The medical student started to sway. "Are you all right?" inquired the surgeon. "I'm just hot," replied Margareta in a faint voice. Counseled by the scrub nurse, she sat down with her head between her legs. The nurse had promptly moved her away from the table, so that if she fainted she would not contaminate the sterile field. Everyone in the OR who had not scrubbed helped remove the student's gown and gloves, and she left the room.

"I guess we know one field she won't go into," I commented. "Not at all. This often happens," said the surgeon. "I should have told her this would happen. I usually do. Then they don't feel bad if it happens, and if it doesn't, they feel unusual. I told you to be nice to her, Sally!" she said in a joking tone to the scrub nurse.

After twenty minutes, Margareta returned. She had scrubbed again, and the nurses helped gown and glove her. As Dr. Adams worked, she described how, when she'd been a student, she'd always been nauseated in the OR. "It's boring if you're not doing it," she declared; she hadn't begun to find surgery interesting and ignore the heat until she had started doing procedures herself. She felt hot right now, she said—she was sweating under her gown, but she was so busy thinking about what she was doing that she didn't notice. Anyone who could just watch an operation without getting bored probably shouldn't be a surgeon, she declared; surgeons find things interesting only when they can *do* something. As she talked, Margareta, who had looked pale and dejected, perked up and began to look rosier and more cheerful. Dr. Adams asked if Margareta was going to come to the lecture she was giving the following month, inviting her to attend. I commented in my fieldnotes: "I think of this approach as the woman's way—not shaming the student, or going into a macho rap about not having the right stuff, . . . but saying of course you get hot and bored when you're not doing anything, and if you get faint, that's just more of the same. Whether or not Margareta ends up a surgeon, she won't have a terrible memory of doing something stupid her first time in the OR."

*Second Vignette.* The surgeon—let's call her Dr. Berman—was observing the intern closely as he worked. She shook her head as he sutured the inch-and-a-half incision in the patient's breast, where she had just removed a lump. She held the thread up with one hand, making it easier for him to stitch. It was obvious that he was having a hard time, but she said nothing, guiding him with her hand. His hand shook and fumbled. I knew she was in a hurry—the OR was running late and she had two more procedures scheduled—but she waited quietly until he had finished, shaking her head in wordless disapproval. The stitches looked scalloped and uneven. They were more proficient, however, than the intern's efforts on the previous biopsy, which had been the first "closing" he had ever performed.

Afterward, when Dr. Berman and I were walking through the winding hospital corridors toward the dressing room, I commented on her silence at the intern's clumsiness. Making him feel bad wouldn't improve his performance, she responded; he'd just get sullen and conclude that he couldn't work with her. "I know what I wanted to say, though," she remarked, as we removed our scrubs and paper-bootiecovered sneakers and donned dresses and street shoes. "My favorite question at such times is, 'What's the matter? First day with a new hand?'"

Surgery has a long tradition of what I think of as "teaching by humiliation." Brutal jokes, aphorisms, adages, and indignities are passed from generation to surgical generation. Neither the victim nor fellow trainees (who inevitably learn what occurred) ever forget such public shaming, and they strive to avoid the "unsurgical" behavior that elicited it.

If teaching by humiliation is a surgical tradition, why did neither woman employ this technique? Why didn't Dr. Adams shame the green medical student, or Dr. Berman pose her favorite question to the maladroit intern? I have never heard a woman surgeon engage in such belittling. Are women calmer, kinder, less choleric than their male colleagues?

Comments by women surgeons support such conjectures. One surgeon believes that "qualities that women in general bring quite unselfconsciously to patient care and resident and student teaching," such as sensitivity, warmth, and compassion, might improve the way surgery is taught, learned, and practiced (Kinder 1985: 103). Two others have declared that male surgeons "are often arbitrary, demanding, and disrespectful," and that "women don't usually command quite as fiercely"—a trait that generates "camaraderie with the other staff members" (Klass 1988). In a more extreme formulation (1986), a woman who chose to remain anonymous compared the "female" operating room with the "male" operating room, contrasting the atmosphere "of peace, tranquillity, and contentment" that a woman surgeon creates to the "tense, hostile, and even explosive" atmosphere generated by a "typical male surgeon."

These sensitive, warm, calm, compassionate women are

surely *doing gender,* behaving in a "feminine" as opposed to a "masculine" way. And such behavior is undoubtedly elicited, encouraged, extorted by the people with whom they interact. But there is more to it than this. I am beginning to believe that some aspects of doing gender in surgery are themselves *embodied.*[2]

Subordinates react differently to male and female bodies in positions of command; these differential reactions are embodied.[3] As Bourdieu notes (1984: 475), "Socialization tends to constitute the body as an analogical operator establishing all sorts of practical equivalences between the different divisions of the social world . . . It does so *by integrating the symbolism of social domination and submission and the symbolism of sexual domination and submission into the same body language*" (emphasis added).

The symbolism, phenomena, values, meanings, and emotions associated with situations where women lead men differ from those associated with situations where women lead women. Naturally, they are closely related. For heuristic purposes, however, I am going to make a somewhat artificial distinction and examine the two types of situations separately.

## WOMEN LEADING MEN

Exploring differences in male and female styles of leadership, I questioned the women surgeons I was studying about their time as chief resident, when they had had responsibility for all the residents under them. Given the structure of the profession, this is the primary opportunity many women have to lead other surgeons.[4] I asked each woman what she had done when she'd encountered a lazy or inefficient subordinate, and how her behavior had contrasted with that of men in similar positions. One described an intern who just hadn't been able to get his work done: he simply did not have the temperament to be a surgeon, and the following year he had switched to internal medicine. She said she had worked with him—would tell him what needed to be done and in what order—and when she'd had time during the day, she would come and help him. When I asked if she had ever seen a man deal with a similar situation, she described how the same intern had dozed off one night in the middle of rounds with a cardiothoracic chief resident.[5] "And he grabbed his tie and he pulled him forward and he said, 'Let me tell you, boy, nobody falls asleep on me unless they're under general anesthesia!'" She'd been "a little more patient" than some of the other chief residents, she said, adding that this had been expected of her: "I think had I said to that guy, 'Nobody falls asleep on me unless they're under general anesthesia,' he would have said, 'Goddam bitch . . . Why can't she find something else to do? Leave me alone.' And it would spread like wildfire among the group, what a cold-hearted woman I was: 'God, she's hard to work with!' That's not my personality, anyway," she concluded, "but I also am smart enough to realize that that's the way everybody else sees it."

A plastic-surgery chief resident described overhearing a telephone call between her fiancé, a chief resident in orthopedics, and a subordinate: "He really let this guy have it." "If I did that,' she said to her fiancé, "he'd be telling everyone what a bitch I was 'cause I yelled at him." She summarized the differences in perception: "The guys telling the guys what to do—it's like the football coach tellin' 'em what to do. And [my yelling] is like the teacher's telling you." A woman's body (integrating the symbolism of sexual and social domination and submission) is out of place in a position of power. This out-of-placeness is manifest to a subordinate man, who reacts to the dominant woman as teacher, mother, "bitch." Her aggressiveness unmans him, returning him to infantile servitude, and her power is chafed against, resented, resisted.

A woman of great power or ability may nevertheless fulfill an alternate embodied role: that of a dominating, terrifying goddess, who must be propitiated for a man to achieve good fortune. The eminent surgeon who was so kind to the green medical student had few difficulties with subordinate men. Some she mentored; others she advised, first-hand or long-distance, on complex problems, techniques, and procedures. Discussing colleagues on her own level, however, she noted: "I think a lot of men are afraid of me, and . . . if you're, if you're, you know, an aggressive powerful guy, those hard—those kind of qualities look good on a guy, and they don't look good on a woman."

A woman chief resident leading young men has no such power. According to the women surgeons, the term "bitch" was used frequently by subordinates to describe a dominant, aggressive female leader. When questioned about her time as a chief resident, Dr. Berman observed: "I think it was also very difficult, at that time and still up until now, for women to behave in positions of authority as regards the junior residents and people junior to them. I believe that most women made a choice of whether to be pushovers or bitches, because there's really nothing in between. There was really nothing in between. And it was difficult to be authoritative . . . in terms of ruling over or directing the actions of men."

Some women explicitly said they had tried male leadership techniques and found them ineffective. Describing how she and her male counterparts had coped with two lazy, difficult subordinates, one woman reported that the men had "screamed more": "When they laid down the law, it was laid down. When I laid down the law, they still thought they could argue." "Did the screaming work better?" I inquired, and she replied, "Not for me." "Did it work for the guys?" I asked. "Yeah, oh yeah," she said. "People shut up and did things. When I yelled, I knew behind my back the one was saying

'Bitch!' and they were both going away complaining how awful I was."

Men have another embodied leadership technique denied to women—what one surgeon called "the buddy-buddy thing." Whenever she had difficulties, she would think about a male resident who had "good authoritative leadership style": "I would say, 'What would Paul do?' . . . And I would try to do what Paul did, and it didn't work! [She laughed.] It didn't work because it couldn't work for me. Because these guys could stand there and say to the junior residents, 'You're embarrassing me. You're embarrassing me—I want you to do this, this, this, and this, and that's it. Period.' And they could somehow, very nonchalantly, toss this off. I just—I couldn't do it!" Both she and the men recognized that she lacked the body, demeanor, manner, and values of a comrade or buddy.

When we examine such embodied knowledge, we are investigating *something that affects the women who lead, as well as the men who are led.* The women have been socialized in the same milieux as the men; they, too, embody the symbolism that conflates sexual and social domination and submission. One chief resident discussed this in terms of self-image. In the tape-recorded interview I conducted with her, she observed that being blunt and impersonal and rather gruff was consistent with the male chief residents' self-image: "In a difficult situation, you need to be in charge and control. You just do it, and it doesn't matter who you rub the wrong way." When I amplified her remark by saying, "Well, it isn't really congruent with your self-image," she responded: "No, I don't want to think of myself as—I guess it's not just my self-image. I get some feedback from the people I work with, and when I perceive that they're, you know, they're unhappy with my behavior, it may be I internalize that too much and say, 'Oh, there's something wrong with me and the way I act. Maybe I shouldn't be this way, maybe I should be—maybe I could get the job done in a nicer way.'" The conflation of internal and external pressures indicates the embodied character of doing gender.

One young surgeon, who noted the psychic and social pressures for her to exhibit more "feminine" behavior ("That's not my personality anyway, but I also am smart enough to realize that that's the way everybody else sees it") managed to work out a "womanly" way to lead subordinate men. When making rounds with younger residents and medical students, she would question them about various tests and measurements: "I would go down to the candy counter and get several packages of peanut M&Ms or somethin' like that. We'd just kind of make a game out of it. Like if somebody knew what somebody's potassium was or what somebody's arteriogram showed, they'd get an M&M or somethin', a piece of red licorice or somethin'."[6]

The more conventionally feminine a woman's demeanor, the closer she came to being a "pushover" as chief resident. "It was the worst year in my life!" declared one remarkably pretty, soft-voiced, feminine woman—whose demeanor I compared, in my fieldnotes, to that of a prom queen and whom I'll call Dr. Carlsen. She reported that some of the residents under her would just take off, leaving unfinished work for which she bore the responsibility. "How did you handle this?" I asked. "I just did it myself," she replied. The body-language of this intelligent, competent, and hard-working woman proclaimed that she posed no competitive threat. Discussing her college years, during which she began to date her future husband, Dr. Carlsen spoke as though her Phi Beta Kappa membership (the certificate was on her office wall) meant little. She said she had loved college: belonging to a sorority, partying, dating her husband-to-be (a surgeon who trained with her), and studying with him and his best friend—who were, she said, much smarter than she was. "I think [it] stretched me, studying with them." She'd had trouble with only one course, organic chemistry (in which she'd earned a B!). Although she had a miscarriage and a baby during her residency, she and her husband finished their training in tandem. Subsequently, she had a second child, and was pregnant with a third, while working part-time as a surgeon (a relatively low-prestige situation). Every word Dr. Carlsen uttered and every gesture she made proclaimed that, although she enjoyed surgery, her main priority was her family.

Compare her description of being chief resident to that of a woman who admitted that her approach to surgery was much like a man's. The conduct and demeanor of this woman, whom I'll call Dr. Deutsch, were not particularly "feminine." Asked how, as chief resident, she handled lazy or incompetent performers, she responded: "Well, I'm a very regimented individual, and I am very single-minded in the way I go about my business, meaning that my way is the right way and there is no other way . . . You do what I tell you, and you don't give me any argument, 'cause if you do, you're going to eat it and I'm going to make you eat it." "How do you make them eat it?" I asked. Dr. Deutsch gave an evil laugh.

> I used to—I was known on rounds to have occasionally brought people to tears by the comments I would make about their ineptitude, about their slackness, things that—I mean, certainly not anything more than telling you bluntly if you are a fool, if you are an incompetent. If I told you to do five things and you did only one or two of them, or you didn't do them correctly and you should have been able to, you will not function well on my service. Or I may shape you up and you may perform better than you've ever performed because you don't want to have another confrontation with me . . . I have a very military, militaristic mindset, and I always did. It's my way or the highway!

The ultrafeminine Dr. Carlsen captivated the senior men who had trained her, several of whom mentioned her with approval and suggested I spend time studying her. While operating, she made two comments about senior men that are indicative of her style. Of one she said, "He tested me for my oral boards. I was scared to death!" Of the second, who had also been one of her examiners, she observed, "He was so sweet!" She had passed her surgery board examinations while doing a year's fellowship after her residency—quite an accomplishment, especially for a woman who was pregnant with her second child at the time. Yet I never felt that her self-deprecating manner was a façade: this was what and who she was. In contrast, Dr. Deutsch, who behaved much like her male peers, neither flirted with nor captivated her seniors. And although her ability has been admired throughout her surgical career, she has paid a professional price for her inability or refusal to do gender.

Superiors might respect a woman's performance and effectiveness as chief resident, while at the same time deploring her "unfeminine" behavior. A woman who had been trained as a family practitioner before entering surgical training laughingly described her year as a chief resident:

> I was relentless when it came to following up on their work, to the point where I got an award for being "whip lady," and then . . . someone said making rounds with me was like making Stations of the Cross! . . . Every year you had to meet with the chief of surgery, and every year I would go in and he'd say, "Any problems?" and I'd say no. And he goes, "Well, you're doing a good job." . . . And my last year, when I was chief resident, the first thing he said to me—he was a guy who likes psychiatry— [was], "Why are you so castrating?" And I said, "what do you mean by that?" "Why are you so castrating that the residents underneath you are *so castrated* when you get done with them?"

Damned if she did and damned if she didn't. She could choose between being castrating and being ineffective.

A few women apparently had minimal difficulties leading male peers. I observed of one chief resident: "She leads quietly, calmly, with apparent confidence, and seems to be followed with no (apparent) challenges from the house officers or students." Subsequently, this young surgeon described how, when she was a child "playing Mass" with her younger brothers, each wanted to be priest; as the oldest of eight children, she got to be priest, while they had to be altar boys. Another, when asked how she related to the men in her training program, responded: "The men in the program I had no problem relating to because I have six younger brothers, so that relating to young men who are somewhat near my age . . . was no problem at all." As a married, pregnant chief resident, the second woman received a special award for exceptional performance. I suspect that neither woman reflected much about leading subordinate men; it was just something each did and had done ever since the first younger brother had become old enough to command.

The inner and outer, the embodied and social constructions of gender reinforce one another. A woman with an authoritative demeanor may have difficulty being an effective chief resident if superiors sabotage rather than support her efforts. A woman who lacks such commanding body language will probably be a pushover no matter what the social context. Chiefs of surgery vary: some encourage women; others take a laissez-faire approach; others are aloof and unhelpful. Thus, one chief resident, after describing the differences between her nonconfrontational leadership stance and that of her male counterpart, a former tank commander in the Israeli army, described a phone conversation she had had with a junior resident a few weeks before: "I was done talking to him and hung up the phone, and he had perceived what I had said, what I had done, as me hanging up on him. And he came out—this is a resident junior to me—came out into the hall and was *very* angry and was yelling at me." In surgery, where chain of command is crucial, this is a significant violation of protocol— rather like an army private shouting at a lieutenant. The chief resident was subsequently called in by the chairman of the department and reprimanded for allowing such a scene to occur. In other words, she, not the junior, was rebuked for his insubordination.

The effect of such lack of support is additive: not only is uncertain leadership further weakened, but the word gets out, making subsequent efforts to exert leadership that much more arduous. The effects of support can also be additive, reinforcing a self-assured stance. What I am saying is that body learning in surgery involves learning not only how to operate on and care for patients, but how to command hospital personnel. Because such learning is embodied, it is more difficult for women to absorb it from men (when, as is frequently the case, no women seniors are present). Social support from senior men, however, makes an enormous difference. A general surgeon described a scene when she was chief resident. I'll quote from my fieldnotes:

There was a patient in the ER [emergency room] whom she wanted to take to the OR. But there was a senior orthopedics resident in the ER who didn't want him operated on and kept holding things up. She went down—she ranked him, she was chief resident—but he was "in my face." "What does that mean?" I asked, and she said he was a big guy, about 6'3", and he was leaning over her and arguing and trying to intimidate her . . . She had been up all night, and was tired, and was hungry, too. And she got so angry she "decked" him. "You did what?" I asked. "I socked him," she explained. In those days, she was even thinner, she weighed about 98 pounds, was 5'2" or so, and she socked this enormous orthopedics resident. Of course, she was called to the chief's office, and he told her she must never hit another surgeon. And she was not allowed to operate for a week—which isn't much of a punishment.

This woman took no nonsense from anyone, ever. This was clearly encouraged by the chief of surgery, who, she reported, acted as her mentor and seemed to have decided it was his special mission to make her, the only woman in the program, into a "surgeon *extraordinaire*." A man can *encourage* a woman to be authoritative, but *body learning* is most easily imparted by other women. When I complimented this surgeon on how well she had run a weekly conference, during which various specialists discussed cases they had in common, she replied, "I've been taught to do that. By a master." The "master" was a woman with whom she had done a fellowship. The "master" did not need to tell her anything about running a conference; this was (as the Japanese term it) *karada te oboeru*—learning or remembering through the body.

I am convinced that learning by body is very close to what psychoanalysts call "identification" and what psychologists describe as "modeling." The results are tenacious, profound, nonverbal. To quote Bourdieu once more: "What is 'learned by body' is not something that one has, like knowledge that can be brandished, but something that one is."

## WOMEN LEADING WOMEN

In 1995–1996 a female surgery resident sent the following query to a column in the *Newsletter of the Association of Women Surgeons*:[7] "I'm running into problems with the nursing staff. They seem to take the other (male) residents' orders without complaint and follow them to a T. But they almost seem to deliberately try to undermine me, going to the attending or chief resident behind my back and asking if what I have ordered should be done for the patient, and so on. What should I do?"[8] Such problems are by no means unusual. Among the women surgeons I studied, some reported no difficulties with nurses, but the subject of female resistance and hostility was frequently mentioned. Young, attractive, vulnerable, sexually unattached women often experienced serious difficulties.[9] Several women reported that they'd had difficulty with female nurses early on, but that this had dissipated over the years. Overall, women surgeons' interactions with nurses differed markedly from those of men.

If we think about sexual and social dominance and submission as *reciprocal* patterns, with one gender embodying dominance and the other submission, then it becomes apparent why a member of the group representing submission has difficulty commanding subordinate women. She has the wrong body. It resembles that of the subordinates.

Discussing nurses, one woman spoke only half-jokingly of the "natural" authority of men: "The nurses . . . seemed to be more willing to accept the natural inherent authority of my male colleagues. They were *much* less likely to accept the authority of women." I would translate this as the *embodied authority* of her male colleagues.

Interactions between surgeons and nurses in the OR are instructive. Examining rituals in the operating room, Katz (1981) analyzes one of the most significant: scrubbing. Scrubbing is precise and beautifully choreographed. The scrub nurse scrubs, dries her hands, and dons her own sterile gown and gloves; she then gives the surgeons towels to dry their hands and assists them in donning their gowns and gloves. Why does the (traditionally) female scrub nurse wait on the (traditionally) male surgeon? Is he incapable of dressing himself? After all, most surgeons are competent and manually dexterous. Does the nurse dress the surgeon because he is busier than she? More important? Or is something else going on, something that is not defined by the dictates of practicality or even sterility? On occasion, I have observed a woman surgeon gown and glove herself, but *never* have I seen a male surgeon gown himself. This aspect of the ritual enacts and helps maintain the traditional relationship between female nurses and male surgeons. The nurses "do deference." In response, the surgeons "do dominance." Like all rituals, it's powerful because it's nonverbal; it is grasped on a bodily, not a cognitive level. (Interestingly, as the world and gender relations change, many nurses are protesting the need to "do deference" in various situations—to be, as they put it, the "doctors' handmaidens.") If the nurses' "rite of sterility" is seen as a way of amplifying the surgeon's greatness, instrumentality, power—in short, his "masculinity"—then it becomes clear why nurses might resent performing this rite, or complementary ones, for other *women*.

The woman who said that female nurses seemed more willing to accept the natural inherent authority of male surgeons added: "They also accepted and went along with certain outrageous behaviors on the part of the men . . . A male colleague, a male resident could blow up and be inappropriate and say terrible things and fifteen minutes later all would be well, and if I—what I felt to be appropriately—threw a tantrum, I would be persona non grata for months." It was universally acknowledged that nurses would punish women who threw "doctor fits" (as the male mentor of one woman termed them). A man who has tantrums is "temperamental" or "high strung"; a woman who has them is a "bitch."

In ten years of studying surgeons, I've seen men throw some spectacular fits. I observed an old-time prima donna scream so loudly and ferociously that he made a young nurse weep; a dry-eyed replacement was quickly furnished. (When this man lost his temper with me once in the OR, I had difficulty holding back my tears.) In the old days, I've heard, an enraged surgeon might actually have hurled a tray of instruments across the room. Yet whenever I heard nurses discuss even the most extreme men, they did so in tones of amusement. Horrified or wry amusement, but amusement nonetheless. The nurses talked about "high-strung" men as though they were naughty, misbehaving little boys who had to be humored, placated, and managed in time-honored female fashion. All the players know the rules to this particular game. These rules are not discussed, or even verbalized; they are something one *does,* not *says.* Assisting a temperamental male surgeon in the OR, the nurses acted as though they were in the presence of a volatile substance that might detonate at any moment; they moved quickly and carefully, attempting to avoid an explosion. The nurses behaved differently with an angry or impatient woman. Another surgeon, who had previously been a nurse, reported: "I think most women learn that if they have a doctor fit they're less likely to get what they want. 'Cause the women, the nurses, will become very passive, passive aggressive, and so you learn other ways to do it . . . You learn quickly. And I think a lot of that has to do with the fact that most of the nurses are women . . . It's men yelling at women versus women yelling at women." A nurse who becomes "very passive, passive aggressive," need not say much. All she has to do is move slowly, hesitate before handing the instruments to the surgeon, or hand over the wrong instrument. This slows the procedure. The longer a patient is under anesthesia, the more danger that patient is in. Women surgeons learn quickly that it behooves them to stay in the good graces of the nurses.

Although I have been told of women who threw tantrums in the OR, I have never observed any. Sometimes I have seen a woman surgeon express impatience to a nurse and then make immediate reparations, explaining in a mollifying tone the importance of a particular maneuver, or why she needed a specific instrument quickly. Once I commented to a transplant surgeon on the fact that she had kept her temper during a difficult time in the OR. She had lost her temper once or twice over the years, she replied, but there had been so many negative sanctions against her that she'd decided it wasn't worth it. In contrast, the tantrums of her male colleague, an extraordinarily "high-strung" surgeon, were a standing joke among the nurses.

In my tape-recorded interviews, I asked each woman what she did if she walked into the OR and found that the instruments she had requested for a procedure were not there (prior to every operation, surgeons fill out cards listing the specific instruments they want the nurses to provide). A chief resident responded: "To lose [your temper] or be direct and demanding rubs a lot of people the wrong way coming from a woman. And so you have to sort of enlist their help, on their level, so that it's not an insult or a demand or an order. But you put it to them so that they participate in the correction of the problem." I said, "So women really do have to behave somewhat differently in these circumstances than men." She answered: "I think sometimes they do. I think . . . where I see it is with . . . women nurses. I actually haven't had a lot of problems with male nurses, personally, when I am in charge . . . The women, not all of them, but some women really resent having me be in charge, or in command, and so you do have to be diplomatic about it." She was not the only woman surgeon to mention that this problem *never* occurred with male nurses.[10]

In response to the same interview question, a senior woman observed: "I probably reacted in ineffective ways. I became angry, resentful, critical, and that usually reinforced the behav-

ior of the nurses. And so, I don't think that's an effective behavior for women surgeons. It's clearly what men do all the
time, but women should not do that with their nursing colleagues." When asked to elaborate on this, she said, "I think
that the nurses, especially in the operating room, and perhaps
in the intensive-care units, are probably nurses that are at a
very high level of achievement, often. And frankly would
rather be doctors than nurses. I suspect that's the underlying
difficulty. And they are very resentful of women who make
demands on them." When asked if she thought the nurses
behave as badly when the surgeon is a man, she replied: "Oh,
no! They are deferential to a fault. They're not deferential to
women, except very very superficially . . . They make [it] quite
apparent that they're being deferential but they don't really
mean it." She laughed and added, "It's quite a tactic!" Women
possess the wrong body for such rituals of dominance and
deference. In return for ritualized enactments of submission,
nurses encourage, elicit, and on occasion extort "feminine"
gender performances from women surgeons. These portray
cooperation as opposed to the domination acted out by the
men. Discussing the behavior of a woman surgeon whom she
obviously liked and had worked with for years, a nurse said to
me: "She *always* brings the stretcher in. She *always* takes the
Bovie pad off. She *always* . . ." She listed other helpful actions
this woman performed that her male colleagues did not. "Always, always, always," insisted the nurse: "Put that in your
book!"

A third woman, who had also been a nurse before becoming
a surgeon,[11] said: "A woman surgeon's leadership qualities
have to [make her] captain of the team as opposed to king of
the hill. And so women surgeons, I think, recognize that . . .
they'll have more trouble than men will trying to exert their
authority through force. And therefore have learned, one way

or another, [that] in order to get the results they need, they have to be the captain of a team and encourage each player to feel their part is important to the workings of the team."

The women I studied had worked out various ways of being captain of the team, as opposed to king of the hill. They were more egalitarian, less authoritarian. They were less hierarchical, treating nurses more as colleagues than as subordinates. They taught more, explaining the reasons for each maneuver and the rationale behind every decision. They were more personal, discussing clothing, children, husbands, home furnishings. In thus doing gender, the surgeons exhibited the characteristics that difference theorists assign to women

I do not wish to suggest that relationships between female surgeons and female nurses are invariably prickly and antagonistic. Nurses can be wonderfully warm and supportive. The older and more demonstrably competent a surgeon gets—and the less the young unmarried nurses perceive her as being a sexual competitor—the more harmonious the relationships may become.[12] I word this in a slightly equivocal fashion because there is some indication that, as women rise in the surgical hierarchy, the rank of the nurses who give them grief also goes up. A senior woman, when asked about her interactions with nurses, responded:

It's not always been a good relationship, and I think that the relationship is somewhat seniority-based. The more senior the nurse, the less accommodating to my considerations that person is. I'll give you some examples. At [she named a department of surgery where she had held a high position], I got along famously with most of the nurses, but not with the nursing supervisor in the operating room, who . . . made it a *point* to make certain that I realized how important she was, and she did not want to accept any of my decisions."

"She resented you," I suggested, and she replied: "She resented, yes, she clearly did. We were about the same age, and I think that she resented it very much. Most of the others, though, were—well, we had very a good relationship, but I think that the more senior the nurses, as a rule, the more equivalent in age, the less able they are to take direction." "From a senior woman?" I inquired. "From a very senior woman." "Well, you know, they meet very few senior women," I observed. "That's true," she said. "And they handle it poorly."

A woman surgeon described the time she had found a Middle Eastern resident near tears: an OR nurse had been harassing her. The resident, whom I'll call Dr. Sahadi, was a quiet, gentle woman, but when she started to talk, a whole history of harassment emerged. Once, when she had been assisting a surgeon from India, the nurse had made unpleasant remarks to the effect that people from the Middle East were incompetent; the surgeon had misunderstood, had taken the reference personally, and had informed her that India was not part of the Middle East. Another time, just before an operation, the nurse had advised the surgeon not to allow Dr. Sahadi to touch the patient; the nurse, who claimed the patient was a friend, said she wanted to make sure the patient got good care. This particular nurse, the surgeon indicated, had gone close to the edge before with many people in many ways. "They're vulnerable," said the surgeon about female residents. "Let her pick on someone her own size, like me." She made up her mind to discuss the incidents with the director of nursing. Later, the surgeon said of the effect such abusive or vicious nurses had on women residents: "They cull out the weak and the sick."

In another hospital, the secretary to the chief of surgery told

Dr. Stephen, the only woman in a surgical training program: "I know why you're here. I know what you did to get here, and what you're doing to stay in this program." Her meaning was obvious: Dr. Stephen had used sexual favors to earn and keep her place in the program.

The women's position encouraged such attacks. Most women surgeons are relatively powerless in hospital hierarchies, making them more vulnerable than men to onslaughts by disaffected subordinates. Female residents are particularly tempting targets: if they complain, they may be branded as weak, whiny females who cannot take the heat. Senior men may subtly, or not so subtly, encourage subordinate women to police other women. The more vicious the assaults, the easier it is for the senior staff members to absolve themselves, observing with mingled horror and satisfaction, "Oh, women are like that!"

The notion of habitus illuminates such incidents. The habitus of Dr. Sahadi, for example, communicated a kind of gentleness and submissiveness utterly different from the independent, self-reliant bearing, tone, and movement of the American women in the training program; a nurse seeking a victim would identify such a woman as fair game. The habitus of Dr. Stephen likewise stood out in her context, which was the Deep South. Raised and educated in a Northern city, she had arrived with husband and children to join a surgical training program which, she subsequently learned, had a history of accepting but not graduating women. She had a bitter and difficult time, but finally succeeded in graduating from the program. (Her experiences are described in Chapter 8.) This surgeon-in-training was clearly the wrong body in the wrong place—a social order where women's bodies had specific movements, meanings, values that were utterly foreign to her. Everything about her was wrong: she was not only a woman, but the first Northerner, male or female, in the training program. I was not surprised to learn that the three women who had managed to finish the program before her were Southerners. Wrong body, yes, but familiar habitus. These three women shared an embodied universe of assumptions with the senior men who trained them. When I outlined the concept of habitus to Dr. Stephen, who was now practicing at a different hospital in the same city, she laughed and mentioned a Southern male surgical colleague who kept telling her, "You don't walk like anyone I know!"

When men routinely do dominance and women do deference, then "the principles of the incarnate social order, especially the socially constituted principles of the sexual division of labor and the division of sexual labor," are unchallenged (Bourdieu 1984: 475). Things are as they were and as they always will be. When, however, someone with *a woman's body* gets out of line, moves out of place, she calls into question these principles of the incarnate social order, thus calling into question the corporeal, symbolic, and social submission of subordinate women. On occasion, subordinates react viciously to such fractures of the embodied social order. This is the dark side of envy: denying their thwarted desire to "do dominance" and their fury at being compelled to "do deference," the women are suffused with murderous rage.[13] The more powerful the target, the more powerful the attacker and the more subtle the attack. Victims are chosen with care; subordinates attack those who seem most vulnerable.[14] *They cull out the weak and the sick.*

# 5 / / / / / / / / / / / / / / / / / / / / / /

# FORGING THE IRON SURGEON

We may abstract from a culture a certain systematic aspect called ethos, which we may define as the expression of *a culturally standardized system of organization of the instincts and emotions of the individuals.*

GREGORY BATESON, *NAVEN* (1936)

The "habitus" transmits from one generation to the next the ethos of groups and classes.

DEREK ROBBINS, *THE WORK OF PIERRE BOURDIEU*

Surgeons tell of a celebrated chief of surgery whose program was so rigorous and time-consuming that the marriage of every surgeon in his department dissolved. According to the legend, the chief and his subordinates were proud of this: they believed that surgery should come first, second, and always. I have not verified the details; I prefer that the man remain legendary.[1] This chief disseminates the vision of what I think of as the "iron surgeon"—powerful, invulnerable, untiring. Those trained by him pass on the mystique, transmitting from one surgical generation to the next an embodied professional ethos. The iron surgeon does battle with death, exterminates disease, declares war on softness, sloth, and error. He is technically brilliant, clinically astute, technologically sophisticated. His feelings, if he has any, are private; his inner life, if he has time for one, is unengaged by his work. The feelings of his patients are also private. Their personalities, problems, hopes, aspirations are irrelevant. The iron surgeon's task is to excise disease. The rest is for nurses or social workers.

This ethos is profoundly gendered. Its values and symbolism are culturally masculine: hardness; cold brilliance; an intense, narrowly focused drive. The mystique of the iron surgeon has limited roles for women: they are cast as patients, nurses, social workers, or disaffected wives vainly seeking tender responsiveness. This is not to say that women never aspire to brilliance and drive, or that a woman cannot be an iron surgeon; they do, and she can. But the meanings, behavior, values, and symbolism associated with the traditional female habitus fit poorly with those of the iron surgeon.

I studied three women trained by a man I'll call James Green, who had himself been trained by the legendary chief. All respected Dr. Green. All feared him. Residents shared stories of his standards, rules, threats, and demands. Surgeons had to change from scrubs to street clothes when leaving the OR suite, even if just for a few minutes. (Many chiefs of surgery allow surgeons to put a "third layer," usually a white coat, over their scrub suits when they leave the OR suite, discarding masks, caps, and paper booties; whereas others insist that true sterility is achieved only by changing clothes. Since changing clothes is inconvenient—especially if one is racing out merely to talk to a radiologist or pathologist, or to grab a quick sandwich from the cafeteria during a lull in a long procedure—such regulations can be hard on surgeons.)[2] Surgeons were not to be seen around the hospital eating, drinking, or even carrying soda or coffee. The women told of a senior surgeon glimpsed from a window, eating a candy bar as he crossed the street; summoned to the chief's office, the man was asked: "Don't you like it here?" They talked of the brutally competitive "pyramid": many began the surgical training program, fewer were permitted to continue, and still fewer ascended to the position of chief resident, thus completing their training at the Temple of Scientific Surgery where Dr. Green reigned. Although a number of surgical programs encourage residents to spend a year conducting laboratory research, this chief exiled some residents to the lab for several years; in this way, rumor had it, he always had extra personnel available in case of illness or emergencies. It was alleged that one unfortunate man had been in the lab for fifteen years (reintegrating a forty-five-year-old resident into a training program poses problems). The terror ran deep. A young surgeon trained by Dr. Green related how, one evening, she was with her husband in a cafeteria, holding a cup of coffee, and looked up to see the chief. Panicked, she thrust the coffee at her husband. "You take it!" she implored. "Jim Green rules by fear," declared a fourth-year resident, worrying that a paper he was presenting at a professional meeting would not meet his chief's lofty standards.[3] The same resident, however, fretted that the interns were not as dedicated as they had been in his day. He thought this might be related to a schedule change—interns were now "on call" every third night instead of every other night—speculating that perhaps the more rigorous schedule selected for the most intense and committed candidates. (Surgical house officers who are on call sleep at the hospital in a special "call room" where they can be reached and awakened for emergencies.)

This is not the only model of surgical training. In 1986 I studied surgeons at a hospital whose chief of surgery, Allen Madison, was universally loved and revered. An excellent surgeon renowned for his technique, Dr. Madison was gentle, warm, and nurturing to subordinates—and indeed to me, when I conducted research in his department. His program had the largest concentration of women and African-American surgical residents I had ever encountered. I suspect that Dr. Madison was celebrated because, among other things, he challenged the dominant surgical paradigm; the legendary chief was celebrated because he epitomized it.

Surgical training is so rigorous, so time-devouring, so stressful, that whether or not the chief rules by fear, candidates invariably absorb some aspects of the iron-surgeon mystique. By the time they have finished their training, surgeons have incorporated a stoic ethos that defies physical weakness and sets them off from the quotidian world. This ethos has been *learned by body*. It is not subject to discussion, analysis, negotiation. It is not something that the surgeon *has*, like knowledge that can be brandished; it is something that the surgeon *is*.

## INSTILLING THE ETHOS

The embodied ethos of surgery involves a denial of the surgeon's bodily needs. This "standardized system of organization of the instincts and emotions," as Bateson puts it (1958: 118), is imparted from the first day of training. The pace is driving, the hours are punishing, and the stakes are terrifyingly high: human lives are in the balance. The intern is on call every second or third night; working through the night does not excuse her from the need to perform well the following day.[4] She is exposed to new techniques that she must master, to statistical outcomes of different treatments that she must memorize, to unspoken rules of behavior that she must obey. This grueling regimen continues for five to ten years, on occasion longer, depending on the surgical subspecialty.[5] Here's how a young surgeon, in a tape-recorded interview, described her schedule during training:

> We were on call every other night. So . . . a typical day or typical two-day stay for me was coming to the hospital between 4:00 and 5:00 in the morning, being there all day, all night, all day the next day, until we went home that evening. And we went home anywhere from 6:00 that night till 10:00 or 11:00 that night, and you were home for four or five hours and then you came back at 4:00 or 5:00 in the morning. And the weekends you had one day off, which could sometimes just be a half a day, depending on how your schedule fell.

Becoming a surgeon involves incorporating distinctive attitudes toward time, food, fatigue, illness, and bodily distress. All are imparted during training; none come "naturally" or effortlessly.

Spending a day with a second-year resident (whom I observed because of the ferocious teasing her hair-trigger "Irish" temper subjected her to), I arrived ten minutes early for the daily 6:00 A.M. rounds. I thus had time to reflect in my fieldnotes on the surgical attitude toward time: "As I waited, I thought about how the training system, with 6:00 A.M. rounds shapes/deforms the character of surgeons. It gives them the habit of rising early; it gives them stamina (through training, and weeding out those who can't make it); and it gives them a particular attitude toward time. It's a bit like the Mad Tea Party: Time will do what I want it to; I will do what is necessary to get Time to do what I want it to do."[6]

The surgical stance toward time and fatigue was contagious: I, too, felt elated and macho when I managed to keep up with a surgeon during a fifteen-hour day. I knew, however, that I could never do this day after day, six or seven days a week, and that I never could have, at any age. Let me quote again from my fieldnotes, when I was observing Dr. Sandra Turner, a chief resident in general surgery:

> I arrived at 6:15 A.M. and left at 9:15 P.M., very tired. But poor Sandy—she [had] left at 10:30 the night before, was tired all day, and also left at 9:15 today, after working far harder than I. And she'll have to be there at 6:30 the next day, which fortunately I don't have to do . . . They have to teach them this stamina young, so that it becomes a way of life, a kind of tunnel vision, so that for the rest of their professional lives, even if they want other things in their life besides work, they still concentrate on their work and their patients and have difficulty "frivoling," or taking time to daydream and gaze at their navels . . . I said something to Sandy, later in the day, about having to learn that stamina young, and she told about her time as an intern, and how punishing it was. She recalled the first time she worked forty hours through . . . She worked forty hours, and had only one meal, and had time to go to the bathroom only once or twice. She lived [near the hospital] then, and walked home to her apartment almost crying. Her feet were terribly swollen. She lay down with her feet above her head, since she knew she'd never get her shoes on if they didn't un-swell. She had only one pair—that is, one pair for work . . . After a while, it wasn't so hard.

One of the things this inhuman schedule is meant to instill (and it generally succeeds) is a surgical superego—an inner voice that compels a surgeon to keep working, despite fatigue, until everything that should and could be done is indeed accomplished. At 9:00 that evening, the exhausted chief resident was ready to leave, when she went to the doorway of the OR to check for the third time on a patient who had just been operated on, first by a team of ear-nose-and-throat surgeons and then by the general surgeons. The patient, who suffered from esophageal cancer, had just had a laryngectomy and an esophogastrectomy. "I'll just go check once more. You don't have to come—you can go home," Dr. Turner said to me, but I followed her. The patient was still on the table, with piles of tubes and equipment on his stomach; the staff was preparing to move him to a bed and the ICU. "Poor little guy," said Dr. Turner, looking at the African-American man, who had been on the table for thirteen and a half hours. He was so pale, he almost looked white.[7] The nurses were so busy counting instruments and needles (which had gotten confused during the long, complex procedure, with two teams of surgeons and several shifts of nurses), that the patient lay there, ignored. "I'm not going to go in [to the ICU], no matter what," declared Dr. Turner, but when I returned from fetching my pen and field-note cards (I had put them away, thinking the day was over), I saw her and the anesthesiologist wheeling the patient to the ICU. "My head hurts," she said to me. But her headache did not stop her from going the extra mile to care for the patient.

Such punishing temporal demands, such highly focused concentration, such indifference to one's own fatigue and bodily discomfort are unnatural for "civilians." They are relatively routine—and utterly necessary—for surgeons. Hunger is one of the bodily needs that must be ignored when it conflicts with the demands of surgery. This, too, is imparted during training. During the thirteen-and-a-half-hour procedure on the "poor little guy," the nurses were relieved for coffee breaks and meals and, when their shift was over, were replaced by another team. The anesthesiologist alternated with two nurse-anesthetists, a schedule that gave each time for coffee, meals, and bathroom breaks. But the ear-nose-and-throat surgeons, who had arrived in the OR at 7:30 A.M., kept working until 5:07 P.M. The general surgeons, who came to the OR at 2:20 P.M., worked until 8:00 P.M., when the patient was finally "closed." Surgeons do not take time off during operations to eat, drink coffee, even to go to the bathroom. Surgical residents learn to eat on the run:

they grab some junk food from a nearby vending machine, keep candy or raisins in their locker, postpone or miss meals. This becomes a way of life.

Another physical sign that must be ignored is illness. The iron surgeon ignores his own pain and bodily distress as far as possible. I made notes on a distinguished senior surgeon who exemplified this stoicism:

> She told me that she had . . . the flu and that she might have to end the day early—she felt really terrible . . . Wednesday [i.e., in two days], she's going to a meeting in San Antonio, and from there is flying back to New York, and from the airport, without going home, [is] flying to Saudi Arabia via Frankfort. Only a surgeon would take it absolutely for granted that she'd go, no matter what. She might end a day early—which she did, at 3:30 (not all that early for ordinary people)—but unless she ended up in the ICU, she'd keep on going, however punishing the schedule, even for a healthy person.

On another day, I observed this ethos being imparted to a fledgling surgeon. An attending physician was teasing the intern for having claimed that he was sick and wanted to leave. Someone had even posted a notice mocking the intern's statement: "I'm sick and am going home." The message was clear: surgeons don't allow themselves to be sick—only civilians are accorded such wimpy privileges.

Such public humiliation is compelling. Once is enough to instill the lesson in the marrow of one's bones: sickness is weakness, and weakness is inadmissible. While conducting research I heard a number of stories about senior surgeons' unsympathetic responses to residents' illnesses. One resident with a fever of 104° attended a departmental Christmas party because she did not want anyone to think she was slacking. When she fainted, the senior surgeons laughed. (The nurse who told the story thought they would not have reacted with levity if it had been a man who fainted.) Another resident suffered gastrointestinal bleeding (a frightening symptom that may herald serious disease) while preparing to scrub on a case. The only thing her chief worried about was who was going to scrub on the scheduled procedure.

I also became acquainted with the results of such indoctrination: women surgeons who were quietly proud of never getting ill, of never taking time off; a resident who worked through the ninth month of pregnancy, by which time she had taken on so much water that her fingers were numb and her stomach was so large she had difficulty reaching the operating table; a Fellow who became pregnant, who broke her leg in a skiing accident, and who contracted Meuniere's disease (which causes dizziness), yet who managed to get to work every day on crutches, to cover for three senior surgeons away at a meeting, and at the same time to write a research paper that won a national award. I was present at an exchange between two women surgeons which illustrated a female version of the iron-surgeon ethos. A breast specialist was scheduled to remove a tiny lump from the breast of her best friend, also a surgeon. After scrubbing, the surgeon entered the OR, where the friend, lying on the table, looked at the surgeon's earrings dangling below the scrub cap and said, "You're in violation of OSHA regulations!" "So are you!" responded the surgeon, looking at the earrings worn by the woman on the table and rapidly getting to work. After removing the lump, assuring her friend it did not feel "gritty," carrying the specimen to pathology (where the lump was diagnosed as benign), returning to the OR, and communicating the diagnosis, the surgeon made an appointment to dine with her friend the following weekend. Neither woman ever referred to the friend's apprehensions. A surgeon feels neither weakness nor fear.

## ASSAYING DIFFERENCES

The experience of being a surgical resident differs for women and men. Some of these differences are extrinsic, based on rules, regulations, and circumstances designed for male residents. Others are intrinsic, based on internalized culture, habitus, and biology.

The female resident stands out: she may be the only woman in the program, the first one accepted, or—even more stressful—the second or third, following others whose performance was evaluated negatively. She is not an ordinary candidate: she represents her sex.[8] Once, during an operation, I heard a senior surgeon conversing with a junior woman:

> He . . . mentioned another woman in the program, Jennifer, who was hated by everyone. She managed to antagonize absolutely everyone there, even patients. Then, at the end, as the final straw, she got pregnant and had a baby. She went off to Atlanta and announced to the people with whom she had just affiliated that she was pregnant again and couldn't take night call. From what [the junior woman] said subsequently, it seems that Jennifer's story was used to tease her a lot. It's more than teasing—it's a kind of warning about what happens to women who step out of line and don't play the game. You'd better make sure you're not a Jennifer.

Not pulling your weight is a serious surgical sin; a surgeon who does not take night call sentences her colleagues to work more nights. Perhaps it is not coincidental that the young surgeon who was cautioned about Jennifer was the pregnant Fellow with a broken leg and Meuniere's disease, who covered for three senior surgeons away at a meeting while writing a prize-winning research paper.

Many programs seem to have a Jennifer-who-did-everything-wrong whose technical, moral, and behavioral errors are used by seniors to warn junior women: *you* had better do everything right. As a woman, culturally defined as weaker and less competent than men, the resident feels people watching, weighing, judging: "If I screwed up, I felt everyone was looking," reported one woman. The trainee may feel overwhelmed by the temporal, intellectual, and emotional demands. Her performance must be better than adequate: she must prove that she is not another Jennifer-who-did-everything-wrong.

Being on call at night is often experienced differently by female residents. At many hospitals, space is at a premium, and women may be expected to share the men's call rooms—even though these may be located in the men's locker room, where the men change their clothes. (Call rooms usually have a bathroom, space to hang coats, and a few lockers where residents can leave their possessions.) When I asked one woman whether she had had special problems as a woman during her training, she sighed, paused, then responded:[9]

> Yeeess. I mean I think, lots of little things and then a couple of big things. One of them, the little things . . . not having a locker . . . When you don't have someplace that you can put your money, when you're on call for forty-eight hours, you have to have some cash around so that you can eat, and if you don't have someplace safe to put it, that's a real hassle. We have no place really to put your clothes . . . And luckily my second year we got a call room for the female surgeons to sleep in, which was very nice. But the first year, I remember sleeping a lot of times on a couch, 'cause the rotation that I was on had a call room but that was in the men's locker room . . . It was just uncomfortable for me . . . The bathrooms were—it was just so unpleasant that it was just easier for me to find a couch someplace to sleep on. Plus, I was so tired most of the time then that I didn't feel like fightin' any more battles about where I was gonna sleep

and what bathroom I was gonna use. It was just easier for me to go someplace else, sleep peacefully for a couple of hours, or an hour, whatever sleep I was going to get—twenty minutes—than it was to have to negotiate with somebody.

These were the "little things." I'll get to the big ones when I discuss abuse.

Female trainees often put social life on hold for the duration. Everyday life itself may be put on hold. A married surgeon rarely sees her husband, and when she does she's exhausted. Married men have the same punishing schedule, but it is taken for granted that a resident's wife will be patient and understanding, care for the children, send his clothes to the cleaners, see that the house is clean, and have dinner waiting when he comes home ready to crash. A husband who provides *any* of these services is considered a saint—or a wimp. Moreover, a husband who does cook rarely takes full responsibility for the food shopping or housework; even the most willing man waits for his wife to tell him what to do, and how. Many women shop for their husband's clothing, but rare is the man who possesses the knowledge and self-assurance to select his wife's wardrobe or to make sure she has clean clothing to put on every morning. In other words, male residents frequently have someone to take up the slack; female residents rarely have such a person. A man who takes up the slack is a paragon; a woman who takes up the slack is a wife, mother, or live-in girlfriend. When asked if surgical training had been as hard for her male colleagues as for her, a young surgeon responded:

> No, I think it was harder for me . . . Probably because they didn't have to try to live their private lives and their residency lives. Their families—usually they were married—would carry that on for them. And they could have the rest of their life just by coming home. And a birthday party would be planned or dinner would be on the table or friends would be coming over for

dinner, so they probably didn't feel as deprived as I did . . . And there weren't just a lot of people to hang around with. I didn't have a chance to meet single women in other fields, and if I met some, my hours were so much worse that there wasn't time to be together. There weren't other single women in my program. And the guys, when they were off, wanted to go out with people that they were romantically interested in or sexually interested in.

The social life of unmarried women residents is often bleak, in marked contrast to that of their male peers. One surgeon said:

Socially, for me, most of the people I knew or hung out with were the people that I met at the hospital. And there was very little other time for [hanging out]. When you got home, you wanted to go to bed. But for [the men] it was different, in that most of the other single people in the hospital their age are nurses that are young women. And so socially it's better for them in that respect. Most of these women tended to cater to them more, and one of my girlfriends that was a medicine intern . . . used to say, "For the guys, it was like being in a candy store." It really was.

I understood what she meant. "All those nurses who dreamed of marrying doctors," I remarked.

Right! And they are—a lot of these guys were not guys you would even look at a second time in another situation . . . I don't mean to be cruel, but they're not—a lot of them are socially immature. Just because the life that we've picked doesn't allow you to mature socially on a lot of scales. And [they] may not necessarily be the best-looking person, and so in other circles people might not perceive them as being desirable. But in this situation, these guys were incredibly desirable and had, you know, three or four or five different people chasing 'em down all the time, wanting to go out with them, and putting little notes in their boxes, and paging them, and bringing them dinner.

Nurses may make life difficult for a female resident whom they perceive as social and sexual competition. A woman who was married during her surgical training told of a friend who was surreptitiously living with her boyfriend. The younger nurses, who were pleasant to the married woman, found occasions to sabotage the work of the one who was apparently unattached.

Unmarried women who date male surgeons frequently make allowances for exhausted residents, but such allowances are rarely accorded women. Said one chief resident:

> I think women will put up with the schedule of a man who is going through his residency . . . maybe for the idea of marrying someone who is going to be making a lot of money in the future—the security or the prestige or whatever of being married to a doctor. Whereas men don't see it that way. I think it's changing, but I think a lot of 'em don't. I think it's very—men like to have somebody to take care of them . . . That's what the one guy that I dated for a long time said: "You're always taking care of everybody else and not me." And it's true. You do take care of other people and not yourself, and not . . . and a man can get away with this.

She talked about the man she had been involved with, a lawyer who was unable to understand her schedule or commitment. She was on a pediatric service and was called almost every night for three months. Somehow she would not be called when *her* family had a social occasion, but every time *his* family had something scheduled, or whenever they were going to meet *his* friends, she would be called and have to go to the hospital. Finally, one evening, when she was called in for a child who had been in an automobile accident, he said, "Don't go. Say you won't come." "I can't do that, you don't understand," she replied. "If you go, it's all over between us!" he declared. "Then it has to be over. I'm going!" she said. That was the end of the relationship. This young surgeon decided that only another surgeon could understand her life, and indeed she eventually married one.

The unmarried female surgeons, then, are surrounded by male peers who are socially and sexually active, while their social lives may be relatively quiescent. The women are less sought-after. In addition, they lack the time to look their best. For a woman, looking attractive takes time: having her hair cut flatteringly, washing it when necessary, selecting becoming outfits, putting up hems, mending and altering garments (or taking them to be mended or altered). "When I was a resident, I lived at the hospital and didn't have time for anything," said one woman, "not even to comb my hair." Such inattention to personal appearance may disconcert a woman who is accustomed to looking, feeling, and being considered attractive.

The grueling five to ten years of surgical training are a woman's prime time for childbearing. Said the woman whose romance broke up over the pressures of surgical training: "I think that's the most difficult, and that's what I always tell medical students or people considering a surgical career: number one, your prime years [are] spent in your residency. Whereas a thirty-two-year-old man can go back and marry the twenty-two-year-old nurse once he's out of his residency, or whatever, and they can have kids for ten years . . . And here I am thirty years old, and during my best years, you know, twenty-five to thirty, I was a resident." In fact, the years spent in training may extend longer than they did for this woman, who at thirty was unusually young for a chief resident.

Some remarkable women do manage to have children and complete their surgical training. For this, they need not only enormous physical and psychic stamina but also support from husbands, chiefs of surgery, peers, and family members. One woman said that when she had been a chief resident she had approached her chief of surgery with the words, "I've got good news and bad news. Which do you want first?" He had asked for the good news, and she had announced, "I'm pregnant!" This had also been the bad news. Fortunately, the chief, like herself, had come from a large, close-knit Irish family and was delighted and supportive. Pregnant surgical house officers are so rare that many programs have not formulated policies to deal with pregnancy: whether women should be given a leave, how long it should be, whether they should be allowed extra time to finish the program. Instead, each case is decided individually, often on the basis of the woman's relationships with her superiors.[10] Peers are often resentful when another resident gets pregnant. If she suffers from fatigue or medical complications, they may wind up with an increased work load, and although they may say little, there may be an atmosphere of bitterness. Thus, one woman, when questioned about problems during her surgical training, responded (with a laugh): "My only problem was doing the extra work for the other female, who was constantly taking maternity leaves. I have fairly strong views about women in surgery, and I don't think women in surgery should have babies." "Ever?" I asked. "Or during their training?" "During their training," she replied. "Because of the amount of extra work it leaves the other residents. And certainly I was on the receiving end of the extra work a lot of the time." Although this woman was more forthcoming than many about her sentiments, the attitude that getting pregnant is somehow a way of dumping more work on one's peers is not rare.[11] Recall that getting pregnant twice was among the sins of Jennifer-who-did-everything-wrong.

A woman who had had her first child as a chief resident and

her second as a junior surgeon said that, in her first academic surgical position, her colleagues had been resentful of her taking time off (she had gone into premature labor and had required four weeks of bed rest) and of the extra call time they had had to assume. Although she had accumulated vacation and sick time, the chief had threatened to cut off her salary: "I pointed out that it was no different than the military leave the men had to take. I said, . . . 'Women have to have babies and men have to go to war, and, you know, the time that I take off is no different than the time you take off for the Naval Reserve.". Taking time off for war, however, is such supremely surgical behavior that it goes almost unnoticed: the iron surgeon is by definition a warrior who engages in hand-to-hand combat with disease and death. Taking time off for pregnancy, on the other hand, is intensely *un*surgical: being pregnant and having a baby designates one's body as that of a patient or wife.

A woman trained in the British Isles described the attitude that had prevailed in the 1980s, during her training: "If you are pregnant, you're virtually unemployable . . . There's the story of Mrs. Gilchrist. Mrs. Gilchrist is a female surgeon in London who had four children, and she did not take any maternity for any of her pregnancies. She worked until the day she had the baby, and then for each child she had, she didn't take any annual leave, but she took all her annual leave at once when she had the baby, and then she came back to work. So that no one could point the finger at her." Here we see a pregnant woman aspiring to the iron-surgeon ethos. But no matter how much strength, stamina, and fortitude Mrs. Gilchrist exhibited, her pregnancy revealed that she had the wrong body for a surgeon, and I suspect many did "point the finger at her." To supremely macho male surgeons, there is something unspeakably disgusting, infuriating, and horrifying about the body of a pregnant woman claiming to be that of a surgeon. As Bourdieu noted, "The sense of distinction . . . which demands that certain things be brought together and others kept apart . . . responds with visceral, murderous horror, absolute disgust, metaphysical fury, to everything which lies within Plato's 'hybrid zone'" (1984: 474–475).

Another problem that is exacerbated during residency (when women are in a particularly vulnerable position) is that of wielding authority: the reactions to temperamental men and temperamental women become even more disparate. I spent a day with Erin Callahan, a second-year resident in neurosurgery whom I met while observing a senior surgeon in her department. When I first encountered Dr. Callahan, I noticed that she stood up for her rights: she complained about the lack of facilities where on-call surgical residents could sleep, and she protested that an intern, rather than herself, should be called to carry out a particular procedure. During this procedure, I also noticed that, unlike the senior surgeon, she did not don spectacles (an AIDS precaution).[12] Dr. Callahan did not do gender with the OR nurses. The senior woman surgeon asked for instruments using a rising inflection: "May I have an extender for a needle?" or "May I have a right angle again, please?" Dr. Callahan, however, merely held out her hand and stated: "Right angle"; "I need a new Bovie—the button on this doesn't work." She seemed like a typical macho surgeon, displaying the kind of behavior that is permitted in men but discouraged in women. I heard from two staff members that the male surgeons gave Dr. Callahan a hard time because of her temper. Indeed, during an operation that I observed, a senior surgeon publicly needled her, saying that her feistiness made her "flaky." In contrast, the chief resident—a man who seemed, if anything, somewhat more arrogant—was allowed to get away with tantrums. It's true that once, when he had caused a scene and thrown a tray of instruments, he'd been reprimanded by a senior surgeon. But I was certain that if Dr. Callahan had dared to throw instruments, she would have been booted from the program.

I characterized Erin Callahan in my fieldnotes as a "social male."[13] Interested in the price that women pay for behaving like men, I asked her if I could spend a day with her. She assented, and at 6:00 A.M. she and I and Dr. Ali Bujra, the chief resident, made rounds together. Dr. Callahan was careful, caring, and conscientious with patients, in contrast to Dr. Bujra, who she told me was called the "Bullet" because of the speed of his morning rounds: he would race into the room, turn on the lights, yank off the covers, examine the patient's incision, often wordlessly, and then leave, without turning off the lights (it was Dr. Callahan who talked to the patients and turned off the lights). Incidents occurred that might have been considered insulting. Once a nurse-anesthetist looked around and inquired, "Isn't there supposed to be a resident here?" When Dr. Callahan identified herself, the nurse said, "Oh, I didn't see you. You're so petite!" Did the nurse not see her because she was small? Or are female surgical residents invisible?

Dr. Callahan and I conversed with a nurse who said she thought women surgeons were different from men—that they were more compassionate. "But they're still surgeons," she added. "They're still perfection-driven." Dr. Callahan said she thought women were more different from men when they began their training than when they finished it: "You're changed," she said, "because of the men who train you." "She's a little fighter," said another nurse about Dr. Callahan. "She sticks up for herself. But they give her a hard time—they ride her." They did indeed, yet it seemed to me that she had a relatively run-of-the-mill surgical temperament: she had a short fuse, stood up for herself, had little patience with incompetence and inefficiency, and was indeed "perfection-driven"—characteristics that would attract no notice in a male resident. As a woman, though, Dr. Callahan was a byword in the department. I heard numerous "jokes" and remarks about her temperament. In contrast, I heard nothing comparable about Dr. Bujra, who, I was told, was not only volatile but misogynistic (referring to all women, including patients, as "bitches"). *His* temper seemed to be taken entirely for granted. Dr. Callahan eventually left the department to enter a training program in a different surgical subspecialty. I cannot know how this decision was related to the way she was treated.

Some women told stories of sexual harassment: a chief resident put his hand inside a junior resident's scrub suit to grope her breast; a senior resident pulled a junior woman into an empty room, where he began to fondle her; a senior surgeon told a resident whom he had favored, "You know, everybody thinks we're screwin' around—we might as well." These were isolated incidents rather than ongoing campaigns, and most of the women seemed to have handled them relatively matter-of-factly: removing the resident's hand, leaving the room, saying no. "They can pitch, but you don't have to catch!" remarked a woman describing one such incident. Other occurrences, involving a *pattern* of inappropriately seductive or sex-related behavior by senior men toward junior women, were more difficult to handle: a chief of surgery made unwelcome advances to junior women, including inappropriate questions about their sex lives; a senior surgeon made scatological remarks and propositioned a young resident in front of co-workers. The more powerful the perpetrator, and the more protracted the campaign of harassment, the more difficult it was for a resident to handle. Incidents of true misogyny were even more serious and frightening. One junior resident (confirming what other women had told me) described assisting a senior surgeon who detested having a woman scrub with him:

> He would stand outside of the room every morning. Nobody liked to scrub with him, so they would put the most junior person on the team in his room, which at the time that I was there was me. And he'd stand outside of the room and scream, "Anybody but the girl! Anybody but the girl! Give me a trained monkey—I'd rather have anybody but the girl!" . . . One day it got so bad that he was stickin' my hand with a surgical instrument! And it's one of those things that you—there's sort of unwritten code in surgery that you don't leave the operating room, you don't leave the bed, you don't leave the patient, and you stand there and take whatever abuse you're going to get because there's sort of this code that you can't leave. . . . Oh, he was—he was bad news. And he had gotten to the point in his career where I don't think he was really very sure of himself, and anybody or anything that he perceived as being threatening—this is the way he handled it. That's finally what I had to keep tellin' myself, because after a while it was more than you could stand. Every day I had to scrub with this guy, for four months.

"What did you do when he stuck you?" I asked. "Well, I moved my hand—obviously!" she replied. "But you stayed in the room?" "Well, yeah, because . . . this guy was a cardiothoracic surgeon and this patient had his chest open and his heart was paralyzed, and . . ." "Every minute counts," I said.

> Right! And me leaving would have left him by himself, which could have put the patient's life in jeopardy. And so you just can't—I mean, you just can't do that. But this particular day it was so bad! I mean, he had drawn blood on my hand—actually, I still have the scars—and the nurse finally said, "Look, I can't take this any more. She has stood here like a Trojan for the last two months and taken this shit"—as she said—"from you, and we've all stood here because you're supposed to be in charge of

this room, but I can't tolerate this behavior any more, and she's done nothing to provoke you!" . . . And she went out and got my chief resident, and he came in and said—pretty much had it out with him in the middle of the case. Told me to leave and that he would finish the case with that guy.

The chief resident knew, from what the nurses had been telling him, that this abuse had been going on for two months, and he finally went to the chief of the department. The junior resident was excused from working with the man, and the department hired an operating-room technician to scrub with this surgeon regularly, so that no other trainees would be subjected to such behavior. The young surgeon concluded the story:

> I can remember the chief [resident] coming in, and he scrubbed in, and I remember lookin' at him, and he winked at me. And I, you know, they were changin' my glove and I was trying not to laugh. At this point, what could you do but laugh? I was trying not to laugh out loud. You either cry or you laugh, and I certainly was not going to cry. And he walked up to the table, and he kind of shoved this guy with his body, and he said, he said, "I look at her like she's a little sister, and I'm not going to stand here . . . even if it gets me fired, I'm not going to stand here and let you treat her like that any more!" And then he looked at me and sort of—he's . . . probably six foot four, huge, your typical sort of stereotype cardiothoracic surgeon, you know, I'm-big-I'm-going-to-save-the-world kind of guy—and he just looked at me and said, "Get out of here!"

It's a wonderful story, with the cavalry coming in to rescue the spirited heroine who had been keeping the villain at bay. The villain, however, remained unpunished; he was merely placed in a situation where he was unable to harass future residents. And the heroine needed assurance from me that neither she nor the other actors would be identifiable in my writings. Such caution is justifiable. The surgical community is small, and the senior personnel who protect abusive men may well punish victims who reveal what occurred. I heard of few such cases of outright abuse. The most serious will be discussed in Chapter 8.

## CULTURE, ETHOS, AND HABITUS

Discussing how she coped with the stress of surgical training, one woman spoke of "things you don't allow yourself to realize until the end." When I questioned what it was that she had not allowed herself to realize, she responded:

> How sick it is to be a surgical resident. It's not even so much a gender thing as just someone so thoroughly controls your life. Actually, "someone" is not even a person—it's just a system, [and it] controls your life so completely, you have no time for yourself. You work endless hours, and you just have to suck it up. You can't ever get mad or show that—not only because that wouldn't be taken well, but because there's nothing you can change. You just have to put up with it. And you know, you miss dentist appointments year after year after year, because you can't ask for an hour off—you can't schedule it. You get so busy that you can't care about people you're taking care of.

This woman was one of the three former nurses in my sample who had attended medical school and become surgeons. It was a grueling, toughening experience. "I spent twenty years, nineteen years after high school, to get my first job—well, the first job that I liked. And there are five years of my life, from general surgery, that are a blur to me. I have very few memories of general surgery . . . and I proved to myself that I have an incredible capacity to tolerate a lot of things."

I believe it is not accidental that this woman, who proved she had an incredible capacity to tolerate a lot of things, was raised as a Catholic. So too was the young surgeon who spent two months standing up to the assaults of the man who wanted "anybody but the girl" to assist him in the OR. In fact, I discovered to my surprise that twenty-five of the thirty-three women surgeons I studied (76 percent) had been raised as Catholics.[14] Although the actual proportion of women studied may not represent the universe of women surgeons, the preponderance of Catholics is surely significant.

On the other hand, only three of the thirty-three women studied were Jewish.[15] I have less confidence in the proportion (9 percent), although it does seem somewhat representative. None of the Jewish women knew of other female Jewish surgeons, and each was surprised because the issue had not occurred to her before I raised it. At the same time, the surgeons and I knew a number of female Jewish *internists* and male Jewish *surgeons*.[16]

Why so many Catholic women? It occurred to me that the Catholic habitus incorporates an ascetic, self-denying embodiment of female achievement: the nun (McNamara 1996: 6).[17] The nun is permitted to obtain higher education, to intimidate and discipline males, and to lead—in the service of humanity.

When asked how she happened to become a surgeon, one woman reported that her greatest influence had been a nun who was her teacher in seventh grade. The nun encouraged students to think about the most important thing they could do, telling them that this was what a woman *should* do. This surgeon's highest term of approbation for a person was to say that surgery was his or her "vocation." In similar fashion, a breast surgeon interviewed by a reporter related how, as the oldest of five children, she had been raised to change the world by doing good work. After joining a convent, she left: the nuns wanted to save their souls, but she wanted to save the world. Discussing the rigors of surgical training, she said: "Most women who survived paid a price: they lost their marriages, or

their minds. I did it by being totally out of touch with myself—
a good old Irish Catholic" (*New York Times*, June 24, 1994: C1).
This knowledge of what it means to be a Catholic woman is all
the more powerful because it involves what one *is*, not what
one *thinks*.

For Catholic women, career options are expanded to include
an austere and rigorous profession which many women consider too harsh to essay. There's a kind of bifurcation, an
either/or quality, in the available options. One Catholic resident, the oldest of seven children, explained: "We didn't want
to be like our mothers."

As a Jewish anthropologist, I found it somehow fitting that
so few Jewish women chose surgery; it made a kind of intuitive gut-level sense.[18] The Jewish women surgeons with whom
I discussed this phenomenon had few explanations. One, who
said she came from a working-class family, suggested that
many middle-class Jewish women are raised to be princesses.
She explained only half-jokingly: "A princess can't be a surgeon—you have to ruin your manicure to scrub!" In fact, none
of the Jewish surgeons I studied could be characterized as a
"princess." (One was the daughter of a professor; another, of a
furrier who died when she was two; another, of an uphol-
sterer.) None seemed to have been overprotected or indulged;
none seemed to expect the kind of financial, emotional, and
social pampering the "princess" stereotype suggests. As I began to reflect on embodiment, ethos, habitus, and surgery, I
realized that these concepts could help account for the scarcity
of Jewish women surgeons.

While conducting fieldwork, I was present during a discussion between two women: a Jewish medical student whom I'll
call Sarah Fisher and an African-American chief resident in
surgery, Dr. Williams. Both were surgeons' daughters. Both
loved surgery. Sarah was trying to decide on a specialty and

was hesitating between surgery and pediatrics, which she was seriously considering. "I don't like the feeling of deferring things," she said. (Discussing the same decision two days earlier, she had mentioned "lifestyle." She was using code words: "lifestyle" refers to time for oneself and family life; "deferring things," to postponing childbearing.) "Don't wait!" advised Dr. Williams, who had just had a baby. She herself had received conflicting advice: the female obstetrics-gynecology residents had told her, "Don't wait!" but the (male) chief of surgery had admonished, "Don't have a baby!" She proposed that Sarah, if she had a baby during her surgical residency, could spend a year doing lab research. Sarah indicated that there were financial pressures: whereas Dr. Williams' husband was an established surgeon and her widowed mother cared for her baby, Sarah's mother lived in a distant city with the student's surgeon-father and Sarah's husband was himself a medical student. Later, Dr. Williams said to me that she thought Sarah had already made her decision: she had opted for "lifestyle," though she was tempted by surgery. Dr. Williams told me that during her recent two-month maternity leave, she had become interested in cooking. She had even telephoned to ask for her mother's recipe for made-from-scratch soup. Her mother had been overwhelmed: "You!" I wondered whether Sarah was reluctant to renounce projects such as homemade soup not only during training but probably throughout her career, and whether the notions of food-as-love and mom-gives-food were particularly salient in Jewish culture.[19]

I found support for this surmise in a telephone conversation with a Jewish woman surgeon, Dr. Bender. She was able to identify only two other Jewish women surgeons, one of whom I had already studied. Dr. Bender didn't dismiss my conjectures about Jewish women's sense of obligation—their feeling that they must cook and care for their families. "I have an eight-year-old daughter," she said, "and I do the standard Jewish-mother things. When I can come home early enough to make fish and broccoli for my daughter, I think I've done a great thing." She paused. "Of course I don't get the time to do it very often." She said she had been unmarried during her training—on purpose. She hadn't thought it possible to be married and go through training at the same time. A friend of hers, a Korean woman surgeon, was experiencing some of the same conflicts between caring for her family and doing her work, and Dr. Bender thought that ethnic background could be a factor in both cases. We both agreed that your sense of obligation to cook for your family is so strong in part because no one tells you you *must* do it; it's something you tell yourself.

Whether or not the "Jewish-American princess" exists (Prell 1990), the stereotype—with its inverse, the "Jewish mother"—is a contemporary American corruption of an ancient embodiment of Jewish womanly virtue. The first attribute of a virtuous woman whose "price is far above rubies" (Proverbs 31: 10–31) is that her husband's heart trusts in her. Female virtue, then, involves marriage and children. *No alternate route exists.* What the virtuous woman *is* is what she *does:* it is her actions, her "works," that earn her the blessings of her children and the praise of her husband. She works "willingly with her hands" to provide food and drink for those in her household and to help the poor and needy; she clothes her family and herself richly; and, by her activity, she supports her husband's position among "the elders of the land." In Jewish ritual belief and practice, the woman in the home is not so much valued as utterly indispensable. Her very body as well as her practices transmits Judaism to her children: she keeps the home ritually pure; prepares meals that observe complex dietary prohibitions; nourishes family, friends, and strangers; furnishes the Sabbath bread, wine, candles, and festive meal; lights the candles to usher in the precious Sabbath "queen" or "bride."[20] Unless a man has a home containing such a woman, it is almost impossible for him to be an Orthodox Jew. The body and practices of the Jewish woman are far more earthy and essential than those of the sentimentalized Victorian "angel in the house": they are simultaneously spiritual and quotidian. This ethos remains when orthodoxy and even religious belief have vanished.[21]

Such a woman has the wrong body for a surgeon. Whether she furthers the interests of her husband and family by working with her hands or by shopping at Bloomingdales, her ethos conflicts with that of surgery. The woman in this body is unlikely to subject herself to five or six ascetic years of training for a profession whose brutal and invasive rituals must, of temporal necessity, supplant the domestic rituals of the Jewish woman.

I am not contending that all Jewish women are imbued with this ethos. Doubtless there have always been some who rebel against traditional values and behaviors (see, for example, Shepherd 1993). Not all Jewish women get married or wish to, have children or wish to, work to nourish and advance the interests of husband and family or wish to. But no habitus exists for Jewish women dissenters. Each must painfully define herself on an individual level as a rebel against an embodied set of structuring principles and common schemes of perception and conception.

I have argued that the iron-surgeon ethos is profoundly masculine. Women can incorporate it—and sometimes this is easier for women with a particular ethno-religious habitus than for others—but there's a price: a price for incorporating the ethos too well, *and* for conspicuously not incorporating it. If—like Erin Callahan or the outspoken chief resident with "a very military, militaristic mindset" we met in Chapter 4—a woman is too "perfection-driven," too arrogant, too *surgical*, her behavior may be resented and punished. If, on the other hand— like the ultrafeminine Dr. Carlsen—she plays down her iron-surgeon attributes, she may be admired by superiors and even male peers, but her "femininity" will jeopardize professional advancement.[22] This double bind occurs throughout a woman's career, but she is particularly susceptible to reprisals during training, just when she is incorporating the iron surgeon ethos.

The double bind is not unique to surgery. Anthropologist Dorinne Kondo noted similar dilemmas in a Japanese workplace: "Women were expected to be appreciative audiences and erotic objects. We women all knew how to play our appropriate identities and thus we participated in the construction of our gender. In so doing, we inevitably facilitated our own subordination" (1990: 297). And again: "A woman at any given moment may feel most comfortable, most accepted, and most integrated into the workplace as she enacts certain familiar, culturally appropriate meanings of gender. At the same time, she at some level surely knows that she is thereby ensuring her exclusion" (1990: 299). Women in the workplace—particularly in embodied vocations that valorize "manhood, manliness, manly courage"—must walk a tightrope. They must incorporate the ethos to do their job well; yet this incorporation must not be so seamless, so successful, that they are punished for being social males.

# 6 / / / / / / / / / / / / / / / / / / / / / / / / /

# THE GENDER OF CARE

> Women, by virtue of the fact that they're women, probably are either maternal or, well, probably mostly maternal, and I think that that's kind of the way you come off most of the time in your relationship, whereas I think men surgeons probably tend to be a little more fatherly, or paternal.
>
> WOMAN SURGEON, IN AN INTERVIEW

Do differences in surgeons' gender have any bearing on patient care? Some of the women I observed were extraordinarily warm, caring, and nurturant with patients. "My role as a surgeon is to try to heal, and part of the healing is caring," said one. These women seemed to conceptualize their task as caring for the *patient*, not just the patient's body (or the parts of the body the surgeon specialized in). Other women, however, paid little attention to feelings, sometimes ignoring not only the psychic but the physical pain caused by their procedures. Observing such behavior, I was often troubled. There was a temptation to sort the women into opposing groups: good/bad, warm/cold, maternal/nonnurturant, compassionate/unfeeling. But this is an oversimplification which obscures rather than illuminates what is going on.

Following are four vignettes from my fieldnotes that show women surgeons relating to patients in a caring, compassionate way. So far as I could tell, being married or a mother did not seem to correlate with such "maternal" behavior. Of the four surgeons depicted here, one woman had four children, one had three, one was married but childless, and one had never married. The first was a general surgeon in an urban setting:

> She was telling me about the poor patients they get at the [surgical clinic]; some of the old ladies look like shopping-bag ladies. She said she always asks them, "How did you get here today?" The answer tells her a lot about the patient's family structure and financial situation. Did a son or friend bring them? Did they take several buses? Some patients do. Did they take a taxi and [get] reimbursed by tokens by the state or city? That happens with some patients. She sounds as though she's really deeply interested in patients' family situations, and plans procedures accordingly: how to schedule a biopsy, etc. She told about a retarded or semi-retarded mother with two semi-retarded daughters she used to see at the Union Health Plan . . . The daughters [had] told [her] in a very matter-of-fact way, when asked about Christmas, that they weren't getting anything because their mother couldn't afford anything. She worries about patients like this, she said.

Now a general surgeon in a small Canadian city:

> We went upstairs to talk to a seventy-year-old man with cancer of the bowel, on whom she's doing a hemi-colectomy tomorrow. He wanted to hear nothing of it—refused to be operated on; he had to take care of his [invalid] wife, he said. He had an enormous hernia; he [had] had it for twenty years and [had] never bothered to have it taken care of. How did you get him to agree to be operated on, I asked. She said she [had] asked him who would take care of his wife the year after next; and then she [had] told him that her dad [had] died of bowel cancer after nine

years; that perhaps he should think of his family, and how they would feel, and perhaps he should discuss whether or not he get an operation with them. The upshot is that he's being operated on, and the son and daughter are taking turns caring for the wife. When she [the surgeon] went into the room, she sat on his bed next to him, companionably, and chatted with him. On the same level, psychically as well as physically. He had to sign a consent form, and when he did something a little tricky, she patted his shoulder and said, "Turkey!" in a loving tone. "You sign better than I," she said, comparing their handwriting. She talked to him the way a loving daughter might.

The third was a breast surgeon in a suburban setting, performing a biopsy on a pregnant patient:[1]

"Things look good in here," the surgeon said to the patient, "really good. Nothing unusual—just normal pregnant breast tissue." The patient said, in an amused tone, "I had a dream last night . . . " The surgeon responded, "The dreams you have when you're pregnant, the erotic dreams of pregnancy—oh, boy!" Both women smiled. The cyst was out and the surgeon said, "I am satisfied that you do *not* have breast cancer, okay? The actual diagnosis you'll have to wait twenty-four hours for, but the reason you're here is to learn that there's no cancer."

The fourth was a hand-and-nerve specialist, explaining what was wrong with a patient and why she believed the problem was not caused by a mastectomy the woman had undergone:

At one point, when she was drawing a particular nerve structure, the surgeon said, with real enthusiasm, "Isn't that neat! I love that kind of anatomy—that's really neat!" The explanation was careful and complete and reassuring . . . The patient, who said she did photography and played an instrument and worried that she [might have] to give both up, seemed to feel much much better by the time the surgeon left. At one point, when the surgeon was explaining to her why she thought the [previous] surgeon [hadn't done] something that injured her, she said a mastectomy is a very boring operation; any operation you do all the time and have no trouble doing is boring—you know just what to do. And if he had touched a nerve, he would have known it—he would have known that something was different. "It's like when you make a peanut-butter sandwich," the surgeon explained to the patient. "Dah, da-dah, da-dah," she mimicked making a sandwich [taking an imaginary slice of bread, opening an imaginary jar and removing something from it with a knife, spreading it on the bread, then taking a second slice of imaginary bread and covering the first one—her movements making it clear that this was one sandwich of many]. "Oh," said the patient, "you mean you'd know if something was different!" The explanation really spoke to her.

The nurturant women encouraged connection. They returned hugs, made little jokes, exchanged rather than merely requested information, mentioning their own families, children, pets when relevant. Like Dr. Krieger the breast surgeon, they gave wonderfully "simple" explanations that even terrified patients with little education could understand. Rather than using specialized information as a scarce resource to reinforce their status, these women shared knowledge; they spent time teaching patients, describing the disease, what could be done for it, what to expect.[2] In lieu of technical terms, they employed everyday images and metaphors—sandwich making, for example. One plastic surgeon, describing the tiny oval cut she would make to remove a mole, compared it to a marquise diamond when she spoke to women, and a football when she spoke to men. These surgeons addressed their patients respectfully by their last name, conversing with them in the same tone of voice they used with colleagues, friends, and residents, rather than the exaggeratedly loud, condescending tone some doctors employ (as though the patient were hard of hearing and dim of understanding). Some women put themselves on the patient's level physically as well as psychically: they sat when talking to hospitalized patients, even if they had to perch on a radiator. I observed one woman kneel when giving bad news to a patient's wife, an elderly woman seated in a chair.[3]

For some women, caring seemed to be fundamental to their self-perception. Describing the difference between the way she related to patients and the way male surgeons did, one woman said: "I think that I'm more empathetic . . . I think that I feel for them more. I think that I have a natural sort of—not compassion, but a natural sort of need to care for people, whereas I think some of my colleagues are very gifted technical surgeons but not necessarily invested in caring for people."

When asked, "Do you think that a surgeon's caring about patients gets them better faster?" one woman responded: "Very much so. On several levels. I think that if there's a bond between the physician and a patient, the patient gets better faster because then they're working together toward a goal. I think if they feel someone is hearing them when they complain, sometimes you just have to complain a little bit and be heard and then you can stop complaining. And I think there just needs to be a certain level of trust, and if you can establish that, then people get well faster. I think it makes an incredible difference."

One surgeon—the woman who said that caring was an essential part of healing, and thus of the surgeon's role—made a distinction between caring about patients and caring "on a personal-dependency level":

> It's probably more a trait of women. That women get their strokes back from patients: "I depend on you and you depend on me—we both need each other. I'm here for you." But that can be a very negative relationship. I think the caring *for* [is important]—as an individual human being, someone I respect but not

as a personal buddy . . . There is the danger of going overboard, and at that point there are always a few patients that one has to find a way to withdraw from and put up the barriers, because patients can become manipulative. And it's happened two or three times where, "You've cared about me—I need you. I'm not going to do well if you're not there for me. I won't do well." I had a woman who told me that if I went to a conference, she'd die. And it was a threat . . . Does one succumb to that threat? [It's] a very difficult thing. And my own reaction [is], if I stay home I have not done her any benefit . . . All I can do is explain that to her—that I hope that when I come back she'll be fine.

Although this surgeon perceived caring as an integral part of her role as healer, she did not allow patients to misuse or abuse her empathy.

Women who were "invested in caring" for people were open and unguarded with patients (and for that matter with me). They did not designate a section of their lives and selves as off limits. A neurosurgeon illustrated this accessibility in an exchange with a cancer patient who was about to be discharged from the hospital: "Can I ask you a personal question?" inquired the patient. When the surgeon assented, she asked, "How old are you?" "Thirty-seven," replied the surgeon. "At first we thought you were younger, and then we decided you had to be older in order to do what you do." "It does take time to be trained," said the surgeon. "You're small, like me. People always think I look younger," said the patient. Both women nodded and smiled. In contrast, a female orthopedic chief resident was much more circumspect. When a patient asked how old she was, the surgeon paused. "Between twenty and forty," she finally responded, in a tone that terminated the questioning. Openness involved expressing empathy and compassion; being guarded apparently closed off these aspects of the surgeon's self.

Thus, whereas some women surgeons cared for and about *persons,* others directed their attention to bodies and disease. I overheard a conversation between a male internist and a female surgeon that exemplified this distinction. They were discussing a patient the surgeon had operated on a few days before. "Fascinating case," said the man. "Metastatic carcinoma all over," said the surgeon. "The organs were all socked in together." "How terrible—poor woman!" said the internist in a pitying tone. But then he cheered up, saying they could present the case at a tumor conference. "The real question," said the female surgeon, "is: *Is it treatable?*" Personalities and pity were not her game. Being a surgeon—the best one possible—was.

Discussing differences between women surgeons and men, Geoff, a Fellow in plastic surgery asserted: "There are two kinds of women surgeons. One kind is motherly—well, maybe that's not the right word." "Compassionate?" suggested a nurse. "Yes, compassionate," he agreed. "She spends more time with patients than the men do, and holds their hands in the OR. The other kind spends less time [with them] than the men. They're one kind or the other, not in-between." A senior woman echoed his distinction. Asked if she related to patients the way men did or differently, she replied:

> I think I relate to them quite differently. I think I'm more sensitive to what they're feeling than the men [are]. Or I listen. I think that a lot of men will see what they're feeling and they will ignore it, because there's no real money in paying any attention to it. And in a way, I can agree with them . . . I will spend a lot of time talking to and evaluating patients, and I know within a minute I am never going to operate on them. I'm not going to make two cents spending any time with them—I should just not have anything to do with them. And I will spend a lot of time listening to them and talking to them about things that basically

are good for them and a waste of my time. I think a lot of men don't want to do that. I just think men don't necessarily like talking about the things that are bothering their patients . . . I think there is a difference between men and women in that re spect.

When I inquired, "So you think that other women also generally relate to patients somewhat differently from men?" she said:

I think they do . . . I think if you looked at the men relating to patients, it would be a normative curve. There would be a very few that would be terrible, a very few that would be superb, and most of them would be sort of average relaters. I think in the women there's actually two curves . . . It's a bimodal curve with the women. I think there's a group that are really—those things that are sort of female qualities of nurturing, mothering, sensitive . . . [But] I think there's a bunch of women that are worse than the average man by far . . . They want to be really macho— more macho than the men . . . You can't believe some of them!

## THE IRON MAIDEN

When surgeons conceptualize their profession as focused primarily on cutting and curing—when they perceive talking to patients as an unavoidable (but not particularly enjoyable) aspect of eliciting symptoms, diagnosing disease, and communicating the need for and results of procedures—then personalities and pity will play little part in their work. Such practitioners are iron surgeons, specializing in action, not words; excision, not empathy. Surgical training instills the ethos of the iron surgeon. And time pressures reinforce a disinclination to communicate with patients: residents must accomplish an almost unlimited number of assignments every day. The task of talking and listening to patients thus ranks very low on the hierarchy of activities valued by their superiors.

Let's observe a hard-pressed chief resident relating to an extraordinarily difficult patient:

During rounds, the chief resident went in alone to see Mrs. Gordon, the difficult old lady, who had a list of questions and concerns for her. She had vomited earlier, and pushed the little tray of vomit toward the chief resident, who quietly recoiled. Clearly, the patient had saved it for her. Later, when the chief resident was talking to the other house officers, she said she thought the woman [had] vomited on purpose; she said she had [had] difficulty not vomiting herself when the woman showed it to her. The young surgeon seemed to think the patient had saved the vomit and showed it to her to harass her, but [a friend of mine in his seventies] says that when he was a child, vomit was always looked at; it was thought that it helped diagnose what was wrong with the patient. Cultural misunderstanding here. In any case, the patient had a long list of concerns; her diet, and the time her meals were served, were one of them. The patient keeps bringing things up, then airily dismissing them. She talked about her diet, then said, "But of course I don't care—I have no appetite." She said in an accusing tone that the dietitian had not visited her the day before, and the surgeon replied, "But you said you didn't want her to come." "Oh, whatever," said Mrs. Gordon in her airy tone, which meant she would put this concern down to raise it the next day. She was worried about a rash on her arm. When she had [had] her colon cancer, she had gotten lots of blood transfusions, and she was worried about the rash, especially since various doctors and medical personnel reacted strongly when they saw it. She had had an appointment with her internist to discuss it, but then she [had gone] to the hospital and couldn't see the internist. What should she do? The chief resident responded that she was an orthopedic surgeon and didn't know about rashes—that the patient would have to talk to her internist . . . When can she see her? How can she make an appointment when she doesn't know how long she'll be in the hospital? inquired the patient. This went on for quite some time. When we left the room, the surgeon said to the other house officers, "I can't do this and run a service—I can't spend all that time. I'm an orthopedic surgeon. I didn't go into this to do social problems!"

This is the kind of patient who would test the forbearance of an older, more experienced doctor. Nevertheless, Mrs. Gordon's concerns were understandable. She had had colon cancer; she was afraid she had contracted AIDS; and she was in the hospital for an orthopedic problem. She was not crazy. The chief resident had had the staff psychiatrists examine her; they'd said she had a depression reaction to her symptoms. Actually, she needed someone to listen to her worries: Did she have AIDS? Would her cancer recur? Would she be helpless from her orthopedic problems? As long as no one listened—as long as the doctors persisted in carving out separate territories of responsibility—Mrs. Gordon was going to keep giving them trouble. Of course, she might have continued to do so, even if they'd listened to her; she was a frightened, sick, lonely old woman. But the chief resident was reluctant to spend time listening. Her concern was to run a difficult, demanding service, seven days a week for four months at a stretch, evenings included. She hadn't been taught that listening was part of her job. She took care of the bones—she was an orthopedic surgeon. Her approach: turf the patient—to the psychiatrists, who could label her "crazy" and invalidate her fears; to the social worker, who could put her in a nursing home where institutional routine would rob her of voice and visibility; to her family, who could ferry her from doctor to doctor in an effort to get her off their hands. An orthopedist did not do social problems, nor did she have the time, energy, and inclination to do compassion. She did bones, like the men who had trained her.[4]

The comment by the young resident Erin Callahan is à pro-
pos here: "You're changed, because of the men who trained
you."[5] The differences that initially set women surgeons apart
from the men gradually diminish. When Erin discussed these
changes, she mentioned a chief resident named Sandy Turner
(whom I had spent time observing): "She was a pussycat when
she began. She's much more bitter now." I once heard Dr.
Turner making what seemed to me like inexplicably brutal
remarks to impoverished patients in the Public Hospital. One
patient, who had just had a breast biopsy, asked when the
results would be available. Dr. Turner said they'd be ready in a
week. "If we don't tell you, ask us. If it's benign, we'll follow
you and see you every six months. If it's cancer, we'll remove
the breast. But there's no use worrying till next week, because
it won't make any difference if you worry." The patient nodded. As if telling her not to worry would prevent her from
doing so!

Why did Dr. Turner, who impressed me as a rather kind,
gentle woman, talk this way to the patient? Had she never
heard a senior surgeon speak differently to impoverished patients? Was it too painful to empathize with a relatively young
woman facing the loss of a breast? Did she just not have the
time to stop, think about the patient's situation, and find a way
to truly communicate with her? Possibly all of the above.
Would Dr. Turner's way of relating to patients alter the following year, when she went into private practice and performed
biopsies on women whose skin color, social background, and
educational level more closely resembled her own? She would
surely have to provide more complete explanations and a
wider range of choices. Would she also offer comfort and compassion? Or had the not entirely benign process of surgical
training changed her irremediably? Had the iron entered her
soul?

Some women absorb the ethos of the iron surgeon all too

well. From "pussycats" they are transformed into pseudo-men. I say "pseudo" because a man who is confident in his masculinity may be able, if he so wishes, to offer comfort and express compassion. A woman who has spent five to ten years learning to *suppress* compassion as "unsurgical" may feel the need to act more macho than the men.

But there's more to it. Surgical training may well change women, but not all women need to be changed in order to incorporate the iron-surgeon ethos. When asked whether women relate to patients the way men do, one surgeon said: "I think that surgery selects out in many cases a group of women who probably have more 'masculine' traits, in that they are assertive, they are aggressive, and [especially] when raised in that tradition that fosters those behaviors. I think if you compared the way women surgeons relate to the way women pediatricians relate, you would find they were not at all similar." In other words, both the ethos *and* the selection process may work in tandem to suppress "feminine" traits.

I'm making it sound as though I agree wholeheartedly with the statement that there are two kinds of women surgeons with nothing in-between. There are surely two kinds. But there are women who fall between the extremes. And there are as many ways of falling between the extremes as there are kinds of human beings. The extremes are visible: some of the women I observed were extraordinarily warm, others extraordinarily cold; some eased the pain of sickness and fear, others exacerbated it. But there were those who seemed relatively impersonal or reticent, and this was how they related to everyone. A woman who did not express warmth freely might be kind to patients, but not particularly empathetic or compassionate. Many seemed to feel that their job was to care *for* patients, rather than to care *about* them. Spending time with various women surgeons, I got the sense that some were warm human

beings, even though they were cool and reserved with patients. Others impressed me as unfeeling. Like a cold man, a
cold woman can be an excellent technical surgeon and take
good care of patients, even if she does not care *about* them.
Some women who seemed relatively cold "faked it": they
asked patients the right questions, but appeared to be observing formalities rather than expressing true personal interest.
It's amazing how obvious the difference was. True warmth and
interest are tangible qualities: one can sense them, just as one
can sense their absence. As psychiatrist Joyce McDougall says
of the mother, "The very timbre of her voice is imbued with her
bodily self and its emotions" (1995: 158). The words that a cold
surgeon utters may be right, but the *music* is wrong. Naturally,
speculations about whether a particular woman is warm or
cold are just that—guesswork that cannot be verified. But observations of various surgeons made it clear that, whatever
their underlying temperament, some women appeared oblivious to the terror and pain of patients and their families.

One young surgeon whom I'll call Dr. Licht—who had previously told me she hated talking to patients—showed a clear
lack of understanding and empathy when she had to explain
to the family of a seriously ill woman that the case was hope-
less. Their mother, Dr. Licht said, was "obstructed" and had
"metastatic disease"; she wanted to "give her a colostomy,"
which would make the patient more comfortable. She stated
that dying of a bowel obstruction was a terrible way to go, but
that since the cancer had "metastasized" there wasn't a chance
of a cure. Naturally, the family had difficulty understanding
any of this. Do many people know what "metastatic" means?
And in this case, of course, comprehension was clouded further by stress and emotion: no one wants to hear that a loved
one is going to die. When a relative of the patient asked
whether the tumor couldn't just be cut out, Dr. Licht's reply

was terse: no, cancers bleed a great deal—"that isn't an option." Afterward, she complained about the family to the nurses: "They live in a whole other world. You should have heard the questions they asked me! They wanted to know why I couldn't cut the cancer out!" Alas, it was Dr. Licht who was living in another world, the world of biomedical science. She didn't seem to understand—or wish to understand—what lower-middle-class patients know or can comprehend, especially when they're worried and frightened.

This is never an easy situation for any surgeon. Conveying bad news to a patient's family is a painful task, and being unable to help a dying patient is frustrating for a specialist whose training has focused on curing, not comforting. The inability to relieve pain and illness is so upsetting that many surgeons refuse to care for patients whose religious principles prohibit transfusions, as was true for the dying woman mentioned above. But although Dr. Licht's reaction may have been born of frustration, the fact remains that it appeared to exacerbate the suffering of the woman's family.

Take, as another example, a general surgeon—Dr. Porter—who practiced in a Canadian university hospital and whom I spent some time observing. In the course of her rounds, we came to the bed of a woman on whom she had done a mastectomy. Dr. Porter told her that she had "found something there" and had had to remove the breast. That was all she said. The patient asked no questions, and Dr. Porter did not stay to see whether she needed any information or reassurance. She made her rounds very very quickly, saying just a few words to each patient.[6]

Dr. Halberstam, a surgical oncologist (that is, a cancer specialist), whom I observed in the operating room during a breast biopsy, was supportive and considerate of the intern she was teaching, while being relatively indifferent to the needs of the patient. During the procedure, the intern performed an injection and Dr. Halberstam alerted the patient: "There'll be a needle stick—going to be a local." (Did the patient understand what a "local" was?) Dr. Halberstam held retractors as the intern made the incision, talking to him in a soft voice. She showed him how to cut the next layer with tiny snips, using sharp scissors. The patient coughed and moaned, but Dr. Halberstam kept going, demonstrating and explaining what the intern should do. It was clear that for her the coughing and moaning were the anesthesiologist's department. When the patient began to retch, Dr. Halberstam advised her to take a deep breath, but it was the anesthesiologist who got something for her to retch into. When Dr. Halberstam started cauterizing the incision, the patient clearly felt it and twice made a sound of great pain. "Gonna be a little more burning," warned Dr. Halberstam, but said nothing to the patient about the pain she had felt. Obviously, this surgeon believed that her responsibility was the *breast;* she left the *patient* to the anesthesiologist.

Yet another example is provided by a breast surgeon, Dr. Dunn, who practiced at a university hospital and whom I spent some time observing. One morning, at about 7:40, we went down to the Ambulatory Surgery holding area, where she met a patient who needed a biopsy. This patient—an attractive black woman—was clearly frightened. She sat in a chair, her eyes enormous. Dr. Dunn, in explaining the procedure to her, used words like "incision" and "suture." I wondered if the woman understood, especially since she was so scared. Dr. Dunn then asked if she had any questions. "I'm a little bit afraid," the patient confided. "Oh, you'll get something to make you sleepy and you'll feel much better," Dr. Dunn reassured her. "Who's your internist? Your blood count is low." "Is that dangerous?" asked the patient. "No," Dr. Dunn replied, "but you should see her afterward. It's not normal." Throughout the interview, I was struck with Dr. Dunn's lack of empathy; she made no effort to touch the patient or to say anything comforting. Again, insensitivity on the part of the physician appeared to aggravate the patient's suffering.

In striking contrast to the four surgeons I have just described was Dr. Carlsen, a breast surgeon who displayed warmth and sympathy toward frightened patients. I observed her examine a woman who had a lump in her breast and whose mother had died of cancer. The patient, who was accompanied by her sister during the examination, confided that she had been up all night worrying. "I can see you're afraid by your eyes," Dr. Carlsen said. She showed the patient the sonogram, explaining why the lump was a cyst and not a cancer. She then asked if the sister wanted to take a look—though seeing a lump on a sonogram, she said, wasn't "as interesting as seeing a baby." Did the patient want her to try to remove the cyst's liquid with a needle?[7] The patient did, and Dr. Carlsen removed the liquid. "Is that all?" asked the relieved patient. "Do you want more?" joked the surgeon. The patient, teary with relief, hugged her, and Dr. Carlsen hugged back. The sister then confessed that she too had been up all night, and as Dr. Carlsen and I left the room, the two women were embracing.

The surgeons I observed were consistent. The same small group of women was responsible for every example I have cited of compassionate, "maternal" behavior. In similar fashion, a smaller group of women was responsible for every example of cold, unfeeling patient care.

The iron-surgeon ethos may suppress or extinguish compassion. But such suppression is neither a necessary nor an inevitable consequence of surgical training. When senior staff members value caring and punish callousness, trainees will take the time and trouble to behave with kindness and respect. Even those who lack compassion can learn to be considerate.

One neurosurgeon described her training program for me, making it clear that consideration was one of the traits it inculcated. Morning rounds began at 5:30 A.M.. If something important had happened in a patient's life that influenced the patient's state of mind (say, the sudden illness of a spouse or child), woe betide the resident who did not know of it. The chief wanted his staff to know *everything* about his patients. When asked to compare her way of relating to patients with the way men surgeons did, the neurosurgeon replied:

> I think I see things that—and relate to patients the same way—the best male surgeons do. I think the surgeons that patients most admire, the male surgeons that patients most admire, are those who are intelligent and technically gifted but who also have a human side. And they see suffering and respond to it, and they see questions and they try to answer . . . I don't think that I'm any better or any worse than the good male surgeons who have been my mentors . . . My role models for the way I relate to patients are men.

"So you don't think women in general relate to patients differently from men?" I asked.

> I think if you were to generalize, and took a hundred male surgeons and a hundred female surgeons, I think you would find that the female surgeons were more capable of responding to suffering and, at least in addressing personal and painful issues, made themselves available to the patients to talk . . . [You would find that they] also considered patient education a more important part of their job, and spent more time answering questions and explaining things.

If such a generalized difference exists (and I've seen evidence that it does), then the more women—the more *compassionate* women—reach positions of authority in surgery, the more trainees, both male and female, will be encouraged to respond to suffering and express caring and compassion.[8]

Any training program whose chief insists on knowing everything about his patients will impart technical skill *and* clinical acumen. Stamina is also underscored: a workday that routinely begins at 5:30 A.M. and that may continue through the following night weeds out softness and sloth. Nevertheless, a chief need not perceive competence and compassion as mutually exclusive. I have heard surgeons speak as though one must choose. Which would you prefer, they inquire, a compassionate surgeon with a good "bedside manner" (a denigrating phrase implying that caring is extrinsic to the surgical enterprise) or a cold, technically brilliant sonofabitch? I see no reason why one must choose. Why not a brilliant *and* caring surgeon?

## "YOU'RE A LADY DOCTOR, SO I CAN TELL YOU"

Thus far, I have discussed the relationship between surgeons and patients as though it flowed in one direction. But the patients, of course, have their own agendas, feelings, actions, reactions. For patients, a woman's body may have a variety of meanings—some overt, others beyond the grasp of words and consciousness; some positive, others profoundly negative.

Women, for example, are expected to be more patient, more sensitive, and more understanding than men. Thus, one patient said to her surgeon, "You're a lady doctor, so I can tell you." She felt fine when she was working, yet when she was doing nothing she noticed all sorts of aches and pains, and she wanted reassurance that this was not unusual. A woman would listen; a woman would understand; a woman would reassure. These expectations are part of the cultural script, whether or not a particular surgeon is indeed caring or compassionate.

To some, a woman's body conveys delicacy and lack of

stamina. Thus, a patient in his sixties agreed to have a female cardiac surgeon perform a coronary artery bypass on him only after stipulating that another surgeon be ready to take over in case she fainted! His wife kept repeating, in disapproving tones, that she had never had a woman doctor; it seemed clear that if she had her way, neither would her husband. On the other hand, I heard another patient, a woman in her sixties recovering from a coronary artery bypass, say to the same surgeon: "I'm very proud to be your patient. I'm very proud you're a woman!"

An eighty-two-year-old woman who had undergone a bypass came to see the same cardiac surgeon for a checkup, and was equally complimentary. "You're a doll!" said the old lady, and responded affectionately to all of the surgeon's directions with, "Okay, doll!" I suspect, though, that however warm her feelings, she would not have taken the liberty of addressing a male surgeon as "doll."

A male patient may simply enjoy looking at a young, pretty doctor. Observing an orthopedic chief resident conduct a clinic at a Veteran's Hospital, I saw her react with a look of annoyance when a nurse reported that an elderly patient had characterized her as "a dance-hall dolly of a doctor!" This was the woman who refused to say how old she was. In contrast, the surgeon who was open about her age accepted comments of this sort with grace and amusement.

These are overt reactions to a woman's body. Other reactions are deeper and less accessible. Said one woman surgeon, "If I tell somebody that these are the things I want them to do, it's sort of like . . . [I'm a] Jewish mother telling you to behave and do these things. And I can be just as firm and just as dogmatic [as a man], but I think that they treat it in the way that they would accept instructions from their mother, who just happens to be a surgeon. Whereas with their male surgeon, they probably accept it with the same fear that they would accept guidance from their father." When patients react to a compassionate, maternal surgeon as though she were a "Jewish mother," they are not aware of why they are reassured by her care and instructions. Their reaction to a woman's body is itself embodied, below the level of words. Such reactions are shaped during the infant's earliest interactions with the mother.

I once witnessed a terrible scene in which a senior surgeon was trying to place a tube in the ear of a struggling, screaming three-year-old as the child shrieked for his mother, who was helping the nurse hold him down. Afterward, I discussed the scene with the chief resident in ear-nose-and-throat surgery. She said she had found a way to make children laugh instead of cry during procedures. She would tickle them on the cheek in front of their ear. When they laughed, she would ask, "Does that tickle?" Then she would tickle their ear, and by the time the tube was inserted they were laughing instead of crying and screaming. Sometimes, she said, she would enter the examining room and immediately begin playing with the child, even before speaking with the mother. "Do the men ever do that?" I asked. No, she said, but children seemed to react differently to men. Whenever she was playing with a child and a male staff member entered the room, the child would start to cry. It was as though they perceived the men differently. Her father had been a surgeon too, and years before, whenever she had assisted him in his office, she'd noticed that children reacted in a certain way to him and another way to her. This surgeon's observations should not surprise us: a woman's body comforts and holds; a man's body acts. A baby learns these distinctions very early; a young child anticipates different behavior from women's bodies than from men's; an adult is impelled by the same embodied knowledge.

The difference in reactions to women's and men's bodies

does not necessarily favor women. Some patients feel less comfortable with a maternal than a paternal surgeon, one who embodies the cultural meanings of fatherhood, even patriarchy. They are reassured by an aloof, commanding, authoritarian surgeon—a godlike, Old Testament figure. I once observed an elderly Italian man kiss his surgeon's hand. I suspect that such a patient would prefer to be treated by a godlike man than a maternal woman, however compassionate.

To some extent, this is a social or *cultural* preference. Patients may also feel a deeper, incommunicable affinity for a man—or, more accurately, aversion to a woman. Experiences with the mother are not always warm and loving; not every mother gives, comforts, holds. To some people, the mother's body represents capriciousness, pain, and betrayal. A motherly surgeon may be anathema to such a patient. Patients may not know why they feel comfortable with one surgeon rather than another, reassured by one body and repelled by another. There are no words to express such embodied tastes and distastes.

Some women, then, are—or are perceived as—maternal. This is not always an advantage, although (as the neurosurgeon said) the surgeons that patients most admire are "those who are intelligent and technically gifted, but who also have a human side . . . They see suffering and respond to it, and they see questions and they try to answer that." Patients admire such surgeons and seek them out.

At the same time, many patients today are unwilling to put up with cold, uncaring, paternalistic care. I met one woman who had come from Denver to Cleveland to have a brain tumor removed. She had gone to Denver to see a world-famous surgeon, who had talked to her for fifteen minutes. In response to her questions, he had told her the procedure was no big deal and that he did it all the time; then he had turfed her to a subordinate to deal with her queries. The surgeons in Cleveland, however, took the time to talk to her as well as operate. The patient was so delighted with her care, that she recommended the Cleveland neurosurgeons to another woman who likewise had a brain tumor and who had received the same sort of insensitive treatment from the surgeon in Denver.

The world is changing; surgery is changing; patients are changing. Charisma is distrusted. "Paternalism" has become a pejorative term. The "white man's burden" that Kipling spoke of is construed by "lesser breeds without the Law" (women, minorities, people of color, oppressed groups, and many patients) as an indictment of white male privilege and empire building. Not surprisingly, cold, remote, paternalistic, godlike surgeons are less in demand.

# 7

## A GREEDY INSTITUTION

> If the norm is male, women will always be the other, the deviant. Superior or inferior, she is not the same. She is caught in a catch-22. If she attacks the problem by trying to be male, she will be too aggressive. If she attacks the problem by trying to be female, she will be the ineffective other.
>
> NANCY A. NICHOLS, "WHATEVER HAPPENED
> TO ROSIE THE RIVETER?"

During a long, lively dinner with a group of women doctors, I inquired whether there was any option for a female professional besides being viewed as a castrating bitch or as an adorable, feminine, slightly lower form of life. "Yes, there is," said one woman. "Mother." We all laughed. She was right, of course. Indeed, each of the stereotyped images currently applied to women professionals has its own problems and double binds.

*"Too Aggressive."* In 1985, when studying general surgeons at a small community hospital, I spent a day with a twenty-nine-year-old Fellow in general surgery. I'll call her Goldie Kline. "She's very outspoken," remarked a senior surgeon. "She tells

attendings [senior doctors] what she thinks of them, and she's alienated some people." Surgery depended on referrals, he said, and since she was going out into practice soon, he wasn't sure it was a good idea for her to be so forthright. He also told me that she was very handy with tools and did all the repairs on her new house. To me, she sounded very much like a surgeon. Obviously, the temperament was not exclusive to men.

Nine years later, Dr. Kline agreed to participate in my study of women surgeons. I was surprised to learn that for the previous eight years, she had been working for a Health Maintenance Organization. Although an HMO is a comfortable niche in today's changing world of surgery, in 1986 it was not the best position for a top-notch surgeon with excellent training. I wondered why she had not been taken in as a potential partner by the most successful surgical-practice group in the community hospital where she had done her fellowship. I had spent time with the exemplary surgeon who led this group and had devoted a chapter of my book on general surgeons to his partner, a compassionate young surgeon. The latter, who was quite critical of surgeons who were less than first-rate, had a high opinion of Dr. Kline's abilities. But instead, the group had taken on a newly graduated resident with rather poor technical skills—a surprising decision.[1] As it turned out, after nine years this young man was no longer with the group; they now had a woman, but it was not Dr. Kline. Through the hospital grapevine, I learned that the new woman was not considered a particularly adept surgeon.

I had observed Goldie Kline operate. She had superb technique and, so far as I could tell, excellent clinical judgment.[2] She had few social graces, however. Dr. Kline was a self-made woman. Her father had died when she was two; her mother had been a seamstress in a factory. She had worked her way through college and attended medical school on scholarships.

She took good care of her patients but had a prickly manner—
she detested having anyone tell her what to do. And she refused to suffer fools gladly. When she thought someone had
done something stupid, she said so in no uncertain terms. In
fact, as a chief resident at a university hospital, she had been so
critical of some young female attending surgeons (whose post-
operative infection rates were, in her opinion, too high) that
they had tried to get her fired.

Goldie Kline spoke, swore, and threw her weight around
like a man—a man surgeon. Here, for example, is her description of a run-in with an anesthesiologist who she believed did
not pay enough attention to his patients:

> My first encounter with him when he came on staff about three
> years ago: the guy spent the entire case on the telephone. Finally,
> after a short period of time, . . . fifteen minutes or so went by, I
> said, "Maury, I want you to come over here. See the head of the
> table? That's where you belong." I said, "You sit your ass on this
> stool. Don't you move until you wake the goddam patient up." I
> said, "I'm not tolerating this crap. You don't have to talk to your
> goddam wife, your stockbroker, or anybody else while we are in
> this room together." And he sat down, and he behaved himself.
> And to this day, I rarely have him on a case.

Goldie Kline drove her red BMW like a surgeon—swerving
in and out of traffic with careless control, adamantly refusing
to let anyone cut her off, exploding at incompetent drivers
who get in her way. "That woman's brain dead. I *hate* women
drivers!"

Not every male surgeon is as profane, undiplomatic, and
outspoken as Dr. Kline. But I remember a general surgeon at
her hospital, in 1985, who had rude manners, a filthy sense of
humor, and dubious ethical standards. He lacked Dr. Kline's
technical proficiency as well. Eventually, however, this man
became chief of surgery at a local hospital. What I am indicat-

ing is that certain kinds of behavior are tolerated—if not exactly welcomed—in a man. A promising but unpolished man will find a mentor who takes him in hand. His wife will join the local women's clubs, make friends with the other elite wives, and help smooth her husband's rough edges. She will select his clothes, decorate and maintain an expensive home, and hold dinner parties to court influential people—who become her husband's patients, refer patients to him, and propose his name for community and medical honors. As every woman surgeon knows, the lack of a wife is a serious handicap.

A promising but unpolished woman, on the other hand, has no one to promote her career, to soothe the feelings of people she may have injured, to work behind the scenes for her success. Her chances of finding a mentor are small. Surgeons who mentor are usually men, and if they take the trouble to mentor women, as some do, they prefer those with charm who make them feel good—women who do gender with flair.

When I told Dr. Kline that I thought if she had been a man with exactly the same characteristics, she would have been far more advanced in her career, she agreed. This intelligent gifted woman was unwilling or unable to do gender. The professional cost had been high.

*The Mommy Track.* Three of the women I studied were salaried;[3] two of these worked part-time. One had two young children and was pregnant with her third; the others had four children each. All were in what colleagues would consider low-prestige, poorly remunerated positions, as part-time employees or, in the case of one, in an unusual practice situation that combined surgery and family medicine.

Two women told of financial promises by surgeon-employers that were subsequently broken. Another, who was pregnant with her second child, told a similar story: the "partner-ship" offered by a former mentor turned out to be permission to share his office space and pay inflated costs for use of the space, facilities, and employees.

Two of these stories sounded like out-and-out exploitation, and the women eventually left. In each case, the woman had relied on the word of a more established surgeon and had joined him—in one case, from another city—without insisting on a written contract. Such trusting behavior may be more common among married women, who may not think of them-selves as primary breadwinners and who may not want to be considered "rude" or "unfeminine": scrutinizing every nitty-gritty detail, arguing vehemently when compensation is in-adequate, insisting on getting every promise in writing, and quitting when a situation is unacceptable.[4] Doing gender puts a woman at a disadvantage; in such a predicament, "feminine" spells victim.

Motherhood does not necessarily make a woman more vul-nerable. I encountered women who had two, three, and four children as well as highly successful full-time surgical careers. Perhaps it is the *intensity of commitment* to motherhood that determines choices. (The intensity of the husband's commit-ment to his wife's surgical career might also affect a woman's options. This will be discussed below.) "You fall in love with those babies!" said one woman, who made it clear that her children came first. "I'm committed to those little lives and helping them become educated adults . . . And if my job gets . . . in the way of that, my job will go without a second thought."[5] Compare this with the attitude of another surgeon, who said: "My priorities are: urgent cares of my patients; and then my family—my children before my husband; and then less important problems with my patients; and then myself."

Another way male colleagues and superiors maneuver a

woman surgeon into the role of "ineffective other" is by characterizing her work as specifically female, and therefore less valuable. Thus, a breast surgeon at a prestigious university hospital inadvertently learned that she was earning $70,000 a year less than a male colleague at the same level; when confronted, the chairman of surgery remarked that what she did was "only titty surgery."[6] She also learned that a similar salary disparity had been a factor influencing her female predecessor's move to another position. Interestingly, male breast surgeons are characterized by their male colleagues as "oncologists" and are generously rewarded for battling the specter of cancer. Needless to say, the work of urologists (primarily men) who specialize in cancer of the testes is highly esteemed; disparaging terms are never applied to procedures on that vital portion of the male anatomy. To a Hemingwayesque surgeon—who glorifies potency and is repelled and terrified at the thought of being placed in a situation of dependency—testicular surgery is a sacrament; breast surgery, a comedy.

*Mother, Wife, Housekeeper.* Men may assume that women do not mind coping with the boring but necessary "housekeeping" details that keep a department of surgery in good working order. One women discussed the pressures on academic women surgeons to take on tasks no one else wanted: "When I took my first faculty job, I joined a faculty with two other men who had started the same year as I did . . . And it became evident to me very rapidly after taking that job that suddenly I was on ten committees, and my colleagues were either not on any or were on one or two. And that a lot of times when there was dirty work to be done in the department, or someone had to get short-staffed, or someone had to do this or that or other things that nobody wanted to do, that person was *me*."[7] The woman resented this pressure and resisted:

It was particularly annoying to me at the level of being a faculty person, because I felt like I had already punched all my tickets. I had proved that I could make it through training; I had gotten my boards; I had done these various things. And this attitude that these guys were part of the club, whereas I had to still prove that I was able to be part of the club, was very annoying . . . Very soon [I started] standing up and saying, "No, I'm not going to do this. I'm not going to be on another committee; I'm not going to be short-staffed. Get somebody else to do it."

Other women, however, do gender and accept such tasks, or at least—in contrast to men—do not protest when they are assigned.

Two academic surgeons I studied took on somewhat traditional female roles in their departments, assuming responsibility for the chores that their high-profile male colleagues disdained. One of them, the only woman in an academic department of surgery, helped the chief make out the monthly on-call schedules and, along with him, took on almost twice as many nights and weekends as her colleagues. Every month she went through the same struggle: the men detested being on call for surgical emergencies, comparing schedules and complaining loudly if they had more nights than someone else. Furthermore, she took responsibility for inserting catheters in cancer patients scheduled for chemotherapy—a small, unchallenging, but necessary procedure avoided by a younger colleague, who, as a new surgeon in the department, should have shared this task but who wanted only the big, important, "interesting" cases that challenged him and won the admiration of his colleagues. She performed the breast procedures that bored the men. She remained silent when another colleague claimed and billed for operations that she herself had performed; since their salary was not based on the number of procedures performed, she allowed him to "hang scalps" at her expense. To me, this woman seemed to fulfill a rather motherly-wifely role: she did what the patients needed, permitting the men to strut, posture, and avoid prosaic tasks. But although she allowed the "boys" their games, she was no victim: when she went to the affirmative-action office to check her salary against that of her colleagues and learned it was significantly lower, she refused to accept the chief's argument that, as a married woman with no dependents, she needed less. She used institutional mechanisms to fight for the raise she knew she deserved, and eventually obtained it.

Another surgeon, also the only woman in her department, assumed responsibility for the bothersome "scutwork" generated by a dynamic, ambitious, charismatic colleague who had so many projects in the works that he could not and would not keep track of the details. She scheduled courses on specialized surgical techniques, teaching them jointly with him; kept track of a book they were writing together, changing materials as his ideas changed, all at peak speed ("either you're first or you're one of the gang," he declared); performed experiments with him, ignoring his mini-tantrums and quietly disagreeing when she thought him wrong; operated with him, as they tried out new procedures. "I don't know—I must be doing something wrong. I can never seem to get my schedule organized," she sighed. "Nonsense!" I protested, pointing out that her high-flying colleague had four women to pick up after him (she herself, his wife, his lab assistant, and his secretary). I told her that I had spent thirty years doing the same thing for an ambitious, charismatic man and that I recognized the scene. When I suggested that the disorganization came from him, she responded quickly: "But there are benefits!" There surely were: with him, she was at the edge of surgical innovation and discovery, and she found her work fascinating. But she was giving up a great deal for these benefits. She was spending so many hours keeping track of the constantly shifting details, that she had little time for a private life.

Being such a second-in-command—anticipating the dynamo's ideas and wishes, shifting direction on a dime when he changes his mind, making her opinions known so gently that he can imagine the impetus came from him—can be a comfortable position for a woman reared to provide a support system for a man. This surgeon indicated that she was not particularly ambitious; she liked the challenge and intellectual stimulation of her work and did not yearn for the worldwide recognition enjoyed by her colleague. Naturally, having such a low-profile woman as lieutenant is comfortable for an ambitious man: he may feel that a junior woman is less likely to scheme to supplant him.

A comfortable position is not necessarily the wisest career choice, however. Not only is such a lieutenant overwhelmed by a host of tedious and constantly changing details, but she is also defining herself, in the highly competitive world of surgery, as in some ways subservient and unsuited to command. As anthropologist Dorinne Kondo has written, "A woman at any given moment may feel most comfortable, most accepted, and most integrated into the workplace as she enacts certain familiar, culturally appropriate meanings of gender. At the same time, she at some level surely knows that she is thereby ensuring her exclusion" (1990: 299).

Does this mean that there are no other choices for a woman surgeon? Must she be defined as a "ballbreaker," as the "ineffective other," or as the mother-wife-housewife who takes responsibility for the details while the boys are busy playing (and scoring points)? I do not believe so. But these are the roles her male colleagues are most likely to accord her. She will probably have to search for and define anything else on her own. There will be little guidance in such a search; she will find few female mentors and role models to illuminate her path. I did, however, meet a number of women who had devised their own ways of being both a woman and a surgeon.

## ALTERNATIVE ROLES

*Respected Associate.* Being second-in-command does not necessarily mean accepting the housewife-mother role, taking care of the details the man does not want to bother with. I spent some time observing Dr. Ann Verdi, a junior surgeon in an academic department, who seemed to have a true partnership with her male mentor. Unlike the association between the meteoric man and the low-profile woman, where I felt the woman was perceived more as a convenience than a person in her own right, this relationship involved autonomy, respect, and harmony. The junior woman took care of details with energy and efficiency but was also encouraged to come up with new ideas and carry them out. So far as I could tell, there was little question of her being perceived primarily as support staff; the senior surgeon cast neither Dr. Verdi nor his wife in supporting roles. He had encouraged his wife to attend law school when their four boys were in high school, mentioning with pride that her schedule as a lawyer was more demanding than his. In similar fashion, he seemed to take pride in the achievements of Dr. Verdi, whom he had helped train. It was clear from their conversation when they operated together that they knew each other well. When they attended meetings, he often brought his wife and Dr. Verdi brought her husband, and there was much badinage about her delight in shopping in the various cities where meetings were held. It seemed to me that he liked having an associate so feminine that she loved to shop and find becoming clothes, and that she enjoyed having a mentor who found this "feminine" characteristic appealing. Dr. Verdi was indeed feminine: she was pretty, coquettish, charming; dressed with flair; spoke of her new husband with romantic ardor; and selected lavender folders for her patient charts, as opposed to the traditional gray ("I wanted an Ann color," she explained). Dr. Verdi was also strong, hardworking, talented, creative, and enterprising. Her mentor was a remarkable man, who apparently possessed so much quiet confidence that he did not need women in a subservient position. She was a remarkable woman, who had been given the freedom to fully express and develop her surgical and administrative abilities. Both benefited from the association.

*Trail-Blazer.* I spent two days observing a senior woman surgeon in her late fifties who held a top administrative position and no longer performed operations. Dr. Anna Swenson's list of honors, awards, consultations, and offices held filled several pages in her extensive curriculum vitae, with an impressive list of "firsts": the first woman elected to membership in a number of prestigious and highly exclusive surgical associations; the only woman ever appointed as chair of a department of surgery at a medical school; the first woman appointed to the editorial board of an eminent surgical journal; and the only woman who has served on an executive body of the most important national organization of surgeons.

When I met Dr. Swenson, I thought she looked just the way a senior—if not *the* senior—American woman surgeon should look. She was tall (at least six feet, I judged, possibly an inch more), had short white-gray hair, and held herself very erect. She was wearing a red blazer, a black pleated skirt, black medium-heeled shoes that looked ladylike yet comfortable, and a lovely white cotton-lawn blouse with a scarf tucked into the neck. No jewelry. She wore enough makeup to look ladylike, but not enough to look as though she were trying to appear seductive or even pretty. Was she pretty? No, not really. Was she plain? No. The categories didn't apply. She was a woman with other things on her mind. She was an attractive person because she was so straight, so evidently honest, and so intelligent. The more time I spent with her, the more attractive and impressive I found her, particularly because she didn't seem to make any effort to impress. She was a commanding presence, without trying to be so. Perhaps her height helped give her this presence; or perhaps it was her moral authority.

Certainly, Dr. Swenson's height was imposing—making it difficult, I suspect, for male colleagues to patronize her ("Now, now, don't you bother your pretty little head about that"). Her manner was not so much "feminine" (which may entail petiteness, cuteness, flirtatiousness, and self-diminishment) as "ladylike." She had a soft voice, which I never heard her raise, and a gentle manner. Well, no, that's not quite right—a *gentlewomanly* manner was probably closer to it. She spoke to everyone—ranging from residents (whom she taught during the day) to me—with warmth and personal interest. Her questions, however, were probing, and it seemed to me that she was someone whom it would be difficult to deceive and impossible to domineer.

In addition to physical presence, Dr. Swenson had moral authority. Honesty and integrity shone from her. She spoke of academic surgery as a calling whose rigorous moral standards she attempted to live up to. She said that for several years she had turned down a promotion to full professor because she did not think she had "reached the proper landmarks." And when I inquired whether her salary as an academic surgeon had been equivalent to that of her male peers, she responded, "Never. Never. From the very beginning until today. It has never been an issue, and I have never made it an issue." When she had been chair of surgery at the medical school and had controlled the salaries, she had always earned less than the others, "even the assistant professors." "And it's . . . almost a matter of principle for me: I don't look upon high salary as being an important factor. In fact, I don't believe that high salary is compatible with an academic career. I found it somewhat repugnant." "You *are* Lutheran!" I commented, knowing her father was a Lutheran minister, and she laughed: "Yeah."

On Dr. Swenson's desk were letters from young surgeons requesting advice; and on the days I observed her at work, she received a number of phone calls from surgeons all over the country, male and female, for whom she was a mentor. One call was obviously from someone getting ready to be interviewed for a job. Dr. Swenson spoke to the woman very frankly, indicating that she really ought to talk to other people about the place, and suggesting some names. "It's a terrible job—I hope she doesn't take it," Dr. Swenson commented afterward. I said that she had talked to the woman very straightforwardly, and she responded ruefully: "I always tell it as I see it. It's the cause of most of the trouble I've gotten into in my life."

During the days I spent with Dr. Swenson, I accompanied her on several errands: to the dry cleaner's, to pick up clothing from one trip that she needed for a second; to the photo store, to pick up color slides from a recent tour; to a fabric store, to pick up a sober, tailor-made outfit that would be appropriate for an upcoming trip to Bahrain (when the clothes were not ready as promised, she quietly said she would return the following day). All were the kind of tasks that I, as a doctor's wife, performed for my husband and that I suspect surgeons' wives frequently take responsibility for. In contrast, the women surgeons I studied took care of their own errands, in person and by telephone. Most were too busy to find, interview, and hire an employee to attend to such details, even if such a person could be located. None of the women surgeons I observed ever requested such personal services from her secretary; several told me they could not and would not, although many of their male colleagues had no qualms about making such demands. One said that her lawyer-husband's secretary did everything for him; he felt that his time was very valuable and that anything a less well-remunerated employee could do to save his time was saving money, including sending his shirts out to the laundry and performing any other personal services he required. In contrast, his surgeon-wife just could not get herself to ask a secretary to do certain things. When I said to one woman (who in fact had an exceptionally helpful husband), "You need a wife," she replied, "That's what we always say: 'We need a wife!'"

Dr. Swenson was the first woman in her surgical training program; in fact, she was the only woman, up to that time, who had applied. When she had been a resident, in the late 1950s and early 1960s, there had been only about 300 women surgeons in the United States.

I studied two other women surgeons in their sixties; each had been the first woman in her training program. One said that until the year she'd been accepted, the booklet describing the program announced that no women need apply; the new chief of surgery who had accepted her application had neglected to mention to anyone that "Dale Lundgren" was a woman! Of these three senior women, two (who were academic surgeons) had never married, and one (who was in private practice) had been divorced twice. Surgery is a consuming profession, and, until recently, few women have managed successfully to combine surgery, marriage, and motherhood.[8]

*Role Model.* At one hospital, in the female surgeons' on-call room, a second-year resident told me how much she was looking forward to working with the celebrated woman surgeon who had arrived at the medical school six months before with her surgeon-husband: "One hundred and sixty articles!" she remarked, in an awed tone. "And she's got four kids, too. And her husband is handsome—he's really cute: I saw him." Dr. Bishop did indeed seem to have everything: a dazzling career, a successful marriage, four children, physical attractiveness, and an imaginative à la mode wardrobe (with up-to-date hemlines). She seemed almost too good to be true. After spending a day observing her, I felt I didn't really understand her. She certainly seemed to have it all—the prizes and achievements, the full professorship, a rewarding family life, a pleasing appearance, an agreeable personality. Her curriculum vitae was seventy-one pages long! And in her spare time, she had co-conducted a survey of women surgeons, asking about their jobs and private lives (the response rate had been 90 percent). A superwoman? She was even nice to her patients!

But my reaction to Dr. Bishop was full of ambivalence, involving some emotions that embarrass me to acknowledge. I wondered whether there was something wrong with me. I rather hoped she would have an Achilles heel. I took her virtues almost as a reproach: it made me feel that I should be more accomplished myself. Her secretary said something to the same effect—that Dr. Bishop's achievements made her feel as if she'd done nothing with her life. I wondered if this was the reaction that high-achieving women always evoked in other women.

I spent more time with Dr. Bishop than with any other woman surgeon, and if she had an Achilles heel I was unable to find it. So far as I could tell, she really *was* brilliant, attractive, kind, decent, happily married, and a caring mother. I mention my initial attitude not because I wish to bare my soul, but because I think this perspective is common among women. We attribute so many of our failures of nerve to gender. When we meet someone who has dared to accomplish—and has succeeded in accomplishing—what we did not even have the courage to attempt or even contemplate, we question ourselves. In trying to find something wrong with the female exemplar, we try to excuse our own deficiencies.

A young surgeon had once inquired, "Elizabeth, how do you do it?" and Bishop had responded, "I'm late for everything—that's how I do it!" Perhaps this is one way she accomplished as much as she did. She also made every moment and every pair of hands count. "You don't have to work day and night," she observed. "You can, if you want to—there's always someone in the hospital to keep you company. But you can get your work done and still have time for a private life, if you wish to do so." She was the only surgeon I studied who put me to work: she said she could not bear to see people idle, and while she did paperwork and made phone calls, she had me collate questionnaire responses. "You'll learn what I'm really like," she declared. "You'll learn what I've been trying to hide from you." Whatever she was trying to hide remained hidden. The more time I spent with her, the more admirable I found her.

Dr. Bishop's curriculum vitae contained an entry I had never seen before—a list of all the students and Fellows she had trained and the honors they had earned. She had conducted her survey of women surgeons in collaboration with a resident, who had received an award for the study. When an article describing the findings was published in a top surgical journal, the resident's name was listed first in the list of authors. When I questioned her about being a mentor, she responded:

> In my career, now, I've never had any problems with anything. No problem at all. But I see now that things are given away, not earned, and I like to give things away to junior people. Like ideas for funding support for something, or cases, or whatever. I like to give them academic presents and teach them: that's giv-

ing stuff away—I like to do that. And I'm very aware when people do that to me. If somebody gives me something, makes me a member of something, puts my name up for something, or promotes me by saying at a meeting we can do this or that, I know what they're doing, and they're being academically very generous. And I've seen it when an academic [is] very selfish, and I don't want to ever do that . . . I do like to mentor. I like to be aggressive about it, I like to be academically generous, and I like to teach my younger guys to be academically generous. And if I see them being selfish, I tell them that. And I tell them they're very bad people: "You are very very selfish. You should be giving first authorship on that paper to So-and-so. He did a lot of work, even if it was your idea." I think what I want to do is populate this country with people who are academically generous, not selfish jerks.

Dr. Bishop went out of her way to instruct female medical students and surgical residents on the best ways of combining motherhood and surgery. During an operation, while demonstrating techniques to a resident, she chatted with a married medical student. "Sarah—that is your name, isn't it?—what year are you in?" she asked. "What are you doing next year?" Sarah said she would get a twelve-week vacation. Dr. Bishop thought that would be a great time to have a baby—she was surprised that all women didn't get pregnant during their residency. When she'd been interviewed for her residency, she'd been six months pregnant. She had borrowed a black dress from her mother and pulled in her stomach. It wasn't that she'd been ashamed of being pregnant, she said, but that she hadn't wanted to make everyone else uncomfortable. By the time she'd begun her residency, she'd already had the baby. Dr. Bishop was the only one I heard offer practical advice on what, to most young women, is a crucial issue: how to be a *woman* as well as a *surgeon*.

What impressed me most about Dr. Bishop as a surgeon was

neither her formidable technique nor her specialized knowledge, but the fact that she had the confidence and compassion *not* to operate when she believed surgery would not help. It was interesting: this world-famous expert spent more time educating patients, and convincing them that they should not have operations unless absolutely necessary, than she did performing operations. This is rare. Most surgeons, male and female, sincerely believe the mock-comic surgical adage "To cut is to cure."

The last day I spent with Dr. Bishop, she held a workshop on her specialty for local doctors. She stood on the stage in front of twenty-five people, looking absolutely comfortable, and lectured without notes from 9:00 A.M. to noon, with short breaks for coffee, and then from 1:00 to 3:00. Her address was on a high level and was packed with information—not one of those dim, dull talks delivered from a basic outline projected on a screen. I felt sorry for the people who trickled in late; they really missed some interesting things. After five minutes, it became clear that she had probably forgotten more about the topic than most people in the audience would ever know. She made little jokes, quoted studies and experiments (some of which she and her colleagues had performed), responded to questions, gave statistics, names, dates. It was a dazzling performance—the kind of lecture where the more one knew, the more one could learn. At the end, she thanked the participants for coming, telling them she had scheduled the workshop because she felt lonesome: she had just moved to town and as yet knew only a few people there. "I need to know people to help me nest in my new city," she said, gesturing unselfconsciously with her arms, hugging herself, showing herself snuggled and nested in a new environment.

In some ways, Dr. Bishop is fortune's darling: it was as though all the good fairies who give gifts had showed up at her christening, while the bad fairy who utters a curse had got the dates mixed and missed the celebration. She worked very hard, as surgeon, academic, wife, and mother, and had achieved a great deal. She did not rest on her laurels, however, nor was her situation picture perfect. The interdisciplinary center for her specialty, promised at the time she'd been enticed from a distant city in 1991, had never been built, and plans for it had somehow evaporated. And unpleasant incidents did occur. I was with her when she gave a talk on her specialty to a group of medical students. The lecture had been scheduled for 11:00 A.M., and when we showed up, the room was in chaos. The previous lecturer, a man in his fifties or sixties, was sitting on the stage surrounded by equipment and conversing casually with students. He paid no attention to the fact that another lecture was scheduled and that it was past 11:00. Dr. Bishop took the microphone, called the students to attention, and began to speak, as the man *very* slowly gathered up his gear. Finally, she stopped and said, "Can I help you do that?" "No," he replied. She calmly waited until he was finished, and then said, "Okay, now that I've got this group to myself, I can start to talk."

It seemed to me that Dr. Bishop had behaved elegantly in response to this man's rudeness. Without displaying anger, she had indicated that she was not going to be pushed around. Her lecture was lively, the slides were provocative, and the students appeared engrossed. As we left, a student entered the auditorium late and said to a friend who had been there, "Looks like fun." "It *was* fun," replied the friend.

A week later, Dr. Bishop received the following letter. A copy had been sent to the chairman of surgery.

Dear Dr. Bishop:

I delayed your lecture to the sophomore class . . . I did not realize, as I was answering questions about the . . . devices which the students were examining, that you were waiting. I apologize that this delayed and visibly upset you.

Should this occur at another time, I encourage you to speak directly to the other lecturer. Beginning your presentation without introduction left everyone flat-footed and dumbfounded. Your statement that I was distracting you as I collected the visual aids was uncalled for.

Faculty should be an example for students. I found your actions rude, and not what I expect from a professional colleague. Your desire to demean me has hurt us both, and sent totally the wrong code for conduct to our students.

The signature was of a piece with the letter: the writer's name was in capitals, with every title and honor he had ever earned listed below. I am convinced that if the recipient had been a man, this doctor would never have sent such a challenging and in some ways mendacious letter. In fact, Dr. Bishop had introduced herself, and had never stated that he was distracting her. (Of course, he also might not have sent it if he had known that an anthropologist was observing and recording the entire exchange!) But a woman who is attractive and relatively young (in her early forties) looks like fair game, and a silver-maned Alpha male may well attack.

Every life and situation has a shadow side, and there was much about Elizabeth Bishop that I did not and could not know. But she was a remarkable and remarkably likable woman who had achieved a great deal, and who went out of her way to help and serve as a role model to medical students and young surgeons.

I met other women, in private practice as well as in academic surgery, who had managed to work out their own ways of being women *and* surgeons. For example, I spent time with one woman nine years earlier, a first-rate technical surgeon who, in the opinion of an older female colleague, lacked the ferocity and drive to succeed in surgery. She had worked for two male surgeons in succession. One had a poor reputation and was not sufficiently successful to keep her; the second was technically brilliant but personally vicious. Eventually, this woman went into solo practice as a breast surgeon, where her gentleness and nurturance were welcomed by patients. They were delighted that—despite having three children and a busy husband, who was likewise a doctor—she was willing to spend hours, in person and on the telephone, calming their fears and discussing the surgical alternatives.

Another woman, Dr. Barucci, who had been trained as a vascular surgeon, could not decide whether or when to have a baby. She'd been far too busy to do it during her fellowship; ditto while she was opening her own practice; then she'd gone into group practice, which hadn't been a good time either; then one of her colleagues, who disliked her, had begun creating terrible problems and objecting to having her made a partner. Finally, after he'd left the practice and the time seemed right, she'd broken her leg! Another surgeon with children told her that no time was a good time to have children: you just have to go ahead and do it. Dr. Barucci was forty and was worried about possible complications due to her age. She was violently opposed to abortion. Whenever she spoke with her best friend, they always went round and round the subject together: Should I have a baby? At last her friend, who was thirty-eight, told her that she'd decided to go ahead. That was it. Dr. Barucci had a thorough physical to make sure she was completely healthy, and then got pregnant. She was sick the entire nine months, lost fifteen pounds, and gave birth to an extremely thin—but adorable and adored—little girl.

Few of these women had the advice and help of older women surgeons. Each had to carve out, through trial and error, a situation that suited her. As more women surgeons succeed in finding their own path, they will serve as mentors and role models for younger women. Every established women I studied made special efforts to help and advise younger women. I saw no instances of what has been called the Queen Bee syndrome, where powerful women discourage younger females, wanting to be surrounded only by lower-ranked men. King-of-the-Hill syndrome among male surgeons, to be sure—but never Queen Bee among the women.[9]

## SURGERY AND PRIVATE LIFE: RECONCILING THE DEMANDS

One of the interview questions I asked was: "How do you reconcile the demands of surgery and those of private life?" There was generally a pause, and frequently a deep sigh. One surgeon responded: "Poorly, I think. I don't have much of a private life." Six others were less direct, but indicated that they, too, had little private life. Some women spoke of priorities and sacrifice, others of setting goals. None made it sound easy. "'Reconcile'? Oh, how do I work it all out? With incredible effort," said one.

Twelve of the thirty-three women surgeons I studied (36 percent) had never married.[10] Several described relationships that ended because of the woman's dedication to surgery. One woman had come close to marrying, but when she and the man had started talking about marriage, he had said: "Of course, you'll retire to take care of the home and children." When I remarked that that was too bad, she said, well, she'd been in love with him, but something had told her it was wrong for her—her heart had told her it was wrong. Her workdays were so hard and her schedule was so full. No man would want to take that on. "It's very difficult for a man to be stood up for the third time in a row because I've gotten called," she said.

Another woman told me she had had a fairly serious romance with a neurosurgeon, but then the two of them had gotten jobs in different cities. And she hadn't wanted to give up her work to stay home and be a "little woman." She had tried dating men both at and below her level of education, but it had never worked out. "What I need is a wife," she declared. "The kind of man who'd be happy taking a secondary role— well, no man would." The relationship with her current boy-friend wasn't really working—she just didn't have the time for him. Whenever he came over, she always had something else she had to do.

Two of the women I studied were divorced. One described how she had moved to a distant city with her husband and given up surgery to care for their two young children. They had had little money, and her husband had been on the road almost all the time for his job. She never knew when he would get home or if he would be home. Her father, a surgeon with whom she had been in private practice, had become ill, and she had commuted back and forth for several years, with the children, to care for him and try to hold his practice together. "That must have been tough," I commented, and she re-sponded: "You do what you have to do, and you do what you want to do, you know." Her husband had finally lost patience, inquiring, "Isn't he dead yet?" The marriage was gradually unraveling. After her father died, she had stayed in her native city and taken over his practice, and the marriage had dis-solved.

Twenty of the women I studied (69 percent) were married. Asked about how she reconciled the demands of surgery and private life, a recently married surgeon said, "I'm still learn-ing." Another, who had several children, replied:

> I don't think you can ever do that. I think you're constantly feeling guilty about both, constantly running around crazy in both environments, and hustling and pushing yourself as hard

as you can in both situations. I don't think there's any neat way you can package it. Just when you think it's packaged, the nine-year-old calls you from the OR and says she's broken her ankle, or is having some disaster; so I don't think there's any way really to control it. My fortune is that there's only twenty-four hours in my day and seven days in my week, and eventually everything gets done that needs to be done and the things that don't get done are usually low priority and don't matter.

One woman declared that behind every successful married woman surgeon is a supportive husband, and that behind every married surgeon who gives up surgery is a husband who does not help. Another was of the same opinion. She had finished two residencies (family medicine, then surgery), had done a year's fellowship in a subspecialty, and then had worked in a hospital emergency room to cover the expenses of opening her own surgical practice. Without someone loving at home, she said, it would have been hard to do it all. Perhaps it is more than "help" that a married woman surgeon needs; her husband must be committed to her being a surgeon.

Surgery is what sociologist Lewis Coser calls a "greedy institution." Surgeons' wives know they must share their husbands. Many were nurses before marrying, and have some idea what they are getting into.[11] Surgeons' husbands must also share their wives—but this goes against the cultural grain. It may be simpler when the surgeon's husband is a doctor, preferably also a surgeon; he will then have some understanding of the demands upon his wife. Whether he is willing to make the personal sacrifices this entails—in not having a traditional wife to take care of his errands, oversee his home and social life, and rear his children—is another question. Five of the women were married to surgeons; five others, to doctors. Two were married to medical researchers, who might be expected to have some understanding of the pressures on their wives. Understanding the pressures, of course, is not the same as a husband's being committed to (and making sacrifices for) his wife's vocation.

Naturally, there are fewer pressures when the couple is child-less. Issues such as who cooks dinner and who cleans the house are elementary compared to the crucial question of who cares for the children and takes primary responsibility for their welfare. Thirteen of the women I studied (39 percent) had chil-dren, and one was pregnant with her first child. These thirteen had one to four children: thirty-one in all. Three women were pregnant when I studied them—one with her first child, one with her second, and one with her third.

I found wide variation in childcare arrangements. Social class seemed to be an issue. One woman sent to England for a live-in nanny; although I did not inquire, I suspect she came from a relatively privileged background and took it for granted that mothers hired competent and, if necessary, expen-sive help to make their lives easier. She gave all her salary to the nanny, who was with the family for nine years. In the surgeon's words, they kept "throwing money at her"; she knew she was the highest-paid nanny around, and stayed. An-other women, who was divorced, had had a Japanese house-man who lived in and prepared meals when her children were young. After that, the family relied on a trusted cleaning woman, who, when the surgeon was called away on emergen-cies, would taxi to the house in the middle of the night and stay with the children until she returned. Speaking of being a surgeon and a mother, she said: "It can easily be done if you've got help, but you've got to have a lot of good help, and it has to be divine intervention. You just don't walk out on the street and find this stuff."

Finding "a lot of good help" to care for household and children is a problem for every working mother; the difficulties are exacerbated for a surgeon, who may have ample funds to hire someone good but insufficient time to find and supervise that person. Frequently, both the surgeon and her husband assume that home and family—including hiring help—are her province. One mother of several children described how her husband, whom she described as extremely supportive, would come to her and say, "How can I help you?" She plaintively observed: "I'd like to tell him, 'Don't ask—just do what needs to be done!'" In some families babysitters cared for the children, who often would be brought by a parent to the sitter's home. Although a sitter is frequently less expensive than a trained nanny or housekeeper, someone else must be hired to clean the house, shop for groceries, do the cooking, and feed the children. One woman placed her baby in the care of her widowed mother; she and her surgeon-husband were building a new house with a separate suite for her mother.

Three husbands took more responsibility than their surgeon-wives for home and children. One had his own business, with flexible working hours. The family had a housekeeper, but he was the one who took the boys to baseball practice and assumed primary responsibility for household emergencies—rushing out, for example, to buy a new washing machine when the old one expired. "Everyone says he's a saint!" said the surgeon's secretary, while the surgeon herself reported that all her friends kept asking if he had a brother. When I asked how she reconciled the demands of surgery and those of private life, she replied: "Well, it takes its toll." "On whom?" I asked. "On both my husband and myself. I think our four kids are thriving. But my husband didn't want a conventional wife . . . or a conventional life, so he doesn't have that." In her opinion, professional women are looking for partners with more education than they themselves have, and they're missing out on some good men.

Another surgeon, who had married a black OR technician, would agree. Black men don't get their identity from the work they do, she said—that's one reason her marriage worked. It didn't threaten her husband that she made more money and had more job prestige than he, nor did it threaten him that she was a strong woman; his mother and sister were strong, and he was used to strong women. When they'd married, they had agreed that when and if she had a child, he would stay home with it. She had, and he did. Both seemed content with the arrangement, and both were starry-eyed about the child, who, the mother was happy to inform anyone within hearing distance, was the most intelligent, most beautiful, most remarkable little girl ever.

The third woman had married a law student when she was in medical school. After finishing surgical training, she had had two children and had been working as an academic surgeon when her husband had lost his highly paid job as a lawyer. Since he had had difficulty finding another, he thereafter stayed home and took on consulting work. Although they had a babysitter who came to the house when the children returned from school, her husband took primary responsibility for household and children. When I asked how her husband felt about her surgical career, she responded:

> I think he's okay with it. You know, when he married me I was just in medical school, so he's been with this since the very very beginning. I think he likes the stories. He loves the stories. He's a real groupie—he's a surgeon groupie . . . And I think he knows that this is really what is good for me, and I think he's okay with it. He's not the kind of person who has a problem with my having a more active career than he does . . . He is a good person. And he's a *decent* person—and I mean that, because not everybody is decent. He is a very decent human being, and an excellent father and parent. His father died a few years ago, but I knew his father, and he's like his father. His father was just a

real gentle soul . . . The rat race was just not for him. He was just a regular guy, and my husband is just the same way—he's just like his father . . . [The] frenetic thing is just not his thing. It's just not.

This surgeon admitted that she was the "crazy person" in the family, and when I remarked that there's room for only one, she agreed. "There is—there really is! I think about that sometimes. I think: What would it have been like if I'd married Bill Gates? Well, it would have been *insane* if I'd married Bill Gates! I mean, he never asked—but you know, . . . it just wouldn't have worked. It certainly doesn't lend itself to a reasonable family life."

She's probably right. Two frenetic, high-strung spouses can lead to fireworks, explosions, and an atmosphere that "doesn't lend itself to a reasonable family life." When one is high-strung and the other calm, they balance each other. Someone is there to pick up the pieces and take care of the details. So far as I could tell, these three women had successful marriages and each considered herself fortunate. And as I made clear to them, I thought they were very lucky. It takes great strength of character to go against the cultural grain; but then, it takes strength of character to be a woman surgeon. As surgeons, these women had proved they could swim against the tide. As wives, they were doing the same.

## BUSHWHACKING

Some of the younger women I spent time with knew no women surgeons with children. I was the one who told them about surgeons I had studied who had managed to combine various surgical subspecialties with motherhood. Questioned about mentors, one woman, pregnant with her second child, responded:

The people that were very important to me—none of them were women. They were all men, and it was a very different example. It was very much a professional example. There were things that they exemplified at different points in my training that I wanted to try to achieve, but there was no one [I wanted to resemble] . . . I wasn't married and didn't have a family while I was in training, but there's never been anyone who prepared me for where I am at this point in my life, [so] that I could say, "Okay, well she did it this way, or she did it that way—maybe I could try that." It's all pretty much blazing your own trail.

This woman was in her thirties. She was keenly aware of the sacrifices she had made to become a surgeon and of the difficulties she was facing in trying to combine motherhood with the practice of surgery. She had no adviser or role model. When I asked whether she would do it again and become a surgeon, she hesitated. "I like what I do," she said, "but I don't like an awful lot of the stuff that goes along with it, and a lot of choices I have to make."

The world is changing; the role of women is changing; and as the number of women in medical school increases, their expectations escalate. Many young women resent being forced to make an either/or choice between a medical career and a family—a choice that men are spared. One prominent academic surgeon, Dr. Travis, told me a story on the occasion of "Take-Your-Daughter-to-Work Day." It seems that her workplace had had a session in which senior women scientists had met with medical students to discuss their careers and the difficulties they had encountered. One of the women, a pediatrician with children, had been transferred to a different city and had begun doing research, since she couldn't practice. She was enjoying a very successful part-time research career, studying important and absorbing problems. At the session, the students had been very interested in what this pediatrician had to say. In contrast, when it had been Dr. Travis' turn to speak, one of the students had said, "But you're not married!"—as though this fact disqualified the surgeon from serious consideration as a role model. Dr. Travis was obviously greatly upset by the student's attitude. That would never have happened when *she* was a student, she said.

As more women enter surgery and blaze their own trails, combining surgery and family life, they serve as role models.[12] Their example demonstrates that it is possible, if difficult, for a woman to have both a private life and a surgical career—that one need not be sacrificed for the other.[13]

I suspect that as the money and prestige associated with surgery diminish and men leave the profession, institutional arrangements will be devised to attract women. These might include not only formal woman-to-woman mentoring, but guaranteed maternity leave and universal leave policies.

I once attended a panel on women in medicine at which a male chief of pediatrics addressed the audience on the "problem" of being pregnant during medical training. Then Dr. Elizabeth Bishop got up to speak. She began by stating that she would like to separate the two *p*'s—"pregnancy" and "problem." Pregnancy, she asserted, is something that is good for the country and good for people. It is not a problem that belongs to the individual woman; she didn't do it by herself or just for herself. Bishop then suggested that the best time for an academic woman surgeon to have children is in medical school and during her training. Being in academia is extraordinarily demanding, and the first three years set the pattern. A woman must produce—she has to do research and write papers; if she doesn't, she will not move forward. Someone should tell young women, Dr. Bishop said, that it's wiser to have their children before then.

There is a lot that someone should tell young women, especially those considering surgery, and mechanisms should be set up so that they learn what they need to know—as do the men. Mentors and role models are vital. I believe they will be provided in the not-too-distant future.[14] Policies that appear impossible when qualified men are available to fill every surgical slot become feasible when the situation changes and women are perceived as desirable candidates.[15] It is not easy to become and be a surgeon. It is even harder to become and be a woman surgeon. But there is no reason that women cannot fulfill themselves both as women and as surgeons. It will always be a balancing act, requiring individual enterprise and effort. But institutional commitment should pave the way. Each woman should not have to bushwhack—to beat her solitary way through impediments—in order to find a path to a satisfying life and career.

# A WORST-CASE SCENARIO

The primary requisite for a good surgeon is to be a man—a
man of courage.

EDMUND ANDREWS, "THE SURGEON" (1861)

Today the Court reaffirms the holding of *Meritor Savings Bank
v. Vinson* . . . "A plaintiff may establish a violation of Title VII
by proving that discrimination on sex has created a hostile or
abusive work environment." The critical issue, Title VII's text
indicates, is whether members of one sex are exposed to disad-
vantageous terms or conditions of employment to which members of the other sex are not exposed.

JUSTICE RUTH BADER GINSBURG, "CONCURRENCE TO
*HARRIS V. FORKLIFT SYSTEMS, INC.*"

It was the weekly "specialty conference" in the Department of Surgery at a Southern university hospital. The residents—all men, with the exception of one woman—were
seated around the table, waiting for the senior attending surgeons to arrive. Every week the same thing happened. Starting
with the chief resident, they would go around the table wordlessly indicating what kind of sex they had had the night before. A tongue flicking back and forth between two fingers

placed in front of the mouth signaled oral sex; a thumb moving in and out of the opposite, lightly clenched fist meant genital sex.

What were the feelings of Dr. Kath Stephen, the lone woman at the table? That boys will be boys and sometimes play rough, and that a girl foolhardy enough to want to play with them has to be confident enough to withstand their boyish braggadocio? This is how the senior surgeons, who set the mood for the department, might have defined the spectacle. Was Dr. Stephen nauseated, as I am when I think of it? Or did she attempt to ignore what was happening and pretend to be elsewhere, as women are said to do when they're being raped? To me, such "games" resemble rape: a group of phallic surgeons-in-training using sex to subdue an unruly female—as is done among some Amazonian and New Guinea tribes, where men punish insubordinate women by subjecting them to gang rape.[1]

Of course, whether or not she admitted it to herself, this young surgeon would have grasped the message before then: that this was not an environment friendly to women. Mothers and wives, yes; *woman* as a category was regarded with veneration and deemed worthy of protection by Southern menfolk. But women who wanted to join the "men's club" were something else. On her first day as an intern, Dr. Stephen had been advised: "Stay away from Pat Hakimian—she's a bitch!" Later she would learn that new women were given the same warning about her. Divide and conquer: the "bitches" fought back; the "pussycats" quit; they did not join forces and confide in one another. During Dr. Stephen's five years of training, six women were accepted and then forced out of various divisions of the surgical training program. Every year, the pressures on her intensified. Only with the behind-the-scenes advice of a lawyer was she able to make it through.[2]

Dr. Stephen managed to finish her training, but the scars

remained. Her once unbounded confidence, optimism, and trust now had limits. These are the qualities which had persuaded her that being a nurse was not enough, that being a nurse-anesthetist was not enough, that being a physician was not enough. She had gone after the most challenging goal of all: being a surgeon. After completing nursing school, nurse-anesthetist training, college, and medical school, she had applied to a surgical-specialty training program at a university hospital in the Deep South.

I must emphasize that I am telling this story as I heard it from Dr. Kathleen Stephen, omitting only a few incidents and details for the sake of clarity. I checked with no one else. The senior surgeons who trained her would surely relate a very different story. Furthermore, my depiction is biased: I empathize with her experiences and sympathize with her distress. Her account makes sense, although this does not mean it occurred precisely as she recounted it. But the weekly conferences—how could she have invented what went on there? In some ways, those poisonous games prefigure everything else that occurred. A department of surgery at a "reputable" university hospital where such behavior is permitted, where such behavior is *generated*, is steeped in misogyny. Such an atmosphere comes from the top; the juniors are merely reflecting what their seniors radiate.

I met Dr. Stephen through a letter. In 1993, when the Newsletter of the Association of Women Surgeons published a brief description of my research, I received letters and telephone calls from women surgeons all over the country who were inviting me to study them. I responded, saying that the National Endowment for the Humanities had cut my requested research funds by a third, and that consequently I could conduct research in only three cities, where I had friends with whom I could stay. Kath Stephen's letter piqued my interest, though. She said that surgery is very different in the South, and that I would learn a lot if I came to stay with her, talk with her women surgeon friends, and observe her at work. I believe that the South *is* in many ways a separate country with a different culture, and I was eager to learn about surgery and women surgeons in the region. Dr. Stephen lived within eight hours' driving distance; if I drove all day to reach her home and then stayed with her, I could afford to observe an area I had never spent time in. I wrote back saying that she had made me an offer I could not refuse and that, when I finished studying women in the three scheduled cities, I would visit her if at all possible.

It was possible, and I did drive there, arriving in mid-afternoon at a large, luxurious, wood-sided house nestled among trees next to a lake. To my surprise, I was greeted by a man, who seemed to be expecting me. That was when I learned that Dr. Stephen was married and had two children. She introduced herself as "Kath," and her husband as "Rafe." She appeared to be in her early thirties, with beautiful bright-blue eyes, short brown hair, and an air of spirit and intelligence. She was barefoot and wore a long sundress. As it turned out, she, like so many of the other women I had studied, had been raised a Catholic. While working as a nurse-anesthetist, she had met Rafe, a radiologist, whom she'd then married around the time she was a student at a prestigious urban medical school. When she was accepted into the Southern program, he had come with her (radiologists can transfer between jobs fairly easily). By now, Rafe had been a full partner in a group of anesthesiologists for four years. This was the only time I lived with the surgeon I was studying. Fortunately, I found Dr. Stephen thoughtful, responsive, and companionable. Her husband was perhaps a bit more difficult, although he seemed anxious to be liked and to win my approval.

The first day I spent observing her at work, Dr. Stephen told me that life was very different in the Deep South. She said that in the South there is a "systematic annihilation of women" who even try to be on the same level as men. Yet Southern men revere their mothers, she continued, describing a lecture given by a world-famous surgeon who had announced that it was his mother's birthday and had asked the audience to stand and sing "Happy Birthday" prior to his talk. I remarked that chivalry and the denigration of women somehow fit together: so long as women were safely isolated on their pedestals, they posed no threat. Southern women—that is, Southern *ladies*— did not become surgeons, Dr. Stephen said. I thought of a woman surgeon I had studied who had graduated from a program in the Deep South; although she had been born in the South, her father had been in the army and she had been raised all over the country. This woman's mother-in-law had been disappointed that her Southern surgeon-son had not married a socialite, and she had probably defined her daughter-in-law as not being a "Southern lady." It could be, I thought, that the pattern or model for such a lady accorded as badly with the role of "woman surgeon" as did the pattern for "Jewish princess": her demeanor, her manners, her very *raison d'être* would conflict with what it took to become and be a surgeon. Not that "Southern ladies" weren't tough, but they didn't *show* the steel—the outer layer consisted of moonlight and magnolias.

In Kath Stephen, one could see the steel. Her intelligence and drive were obvious; she made no attempt to cover them with a little-woman veneer. This was the drive that had propelled her, the oldest of six children from a lower-middle-class family, into a career as a surgeon. She described the progression: "I started out as a nurse. My mother was a nurse, and it was the highest thing I felt I could aspire to at that time. After going through nursing school, I realized that I wanted more;

and given the horizons I had at the time, I felt that the most I could do was be a nurse-anesthetist. So I went through nurse-anesthesia school and got my first job . . . That was the first real exposure I had to physicians as people and what they actually knew, and I realized at that time that I can do this!"[3] When she went to school to become a nurse-anesthetist, her fireman-father had inquired, "When are you going to stop going to school and get a real job?" while her mother had complained, "I won't be able to talk to you—I won't be able to talk to you at all." Clearly, she had done it on her own, with no encouragement from her family. When I asked how it had happened that she'd become a surgeon, she said:

> I went to medical school thinking that I'd go into anesthesia, because I loved being a nurse-anesthetist . . . I had watched surgeons for a number of years . . . I was *extremely* sensitive to the way they were—the devil-may-care, the arrogance, the forceful dominant nature of the lot of them—and was hesitant to go into surgery. I liked working with my hands . . . so I knew that I would like surgery. The question was: Did I have to be one of these personalities to be a surgeon? . . . I was able to make that decision only after working at [a high-level government health agency], which was part of my job as a nurse-anesthetist . . . I spent a year at [the agency] in the operating rooms as a nurse-anesthetist, and it was only there that I saw that surgeons didn't have to be arrogant, uh, assholes. [She laughed.] These men cared for their patients. They were thoughtful, they were careful, they were well-balanced, they listened, and they cared for their patients—in addition to being decisive and technically good. They were scientific in their thinking, they were interested in research, they were interested in contributing to the common good. They weren't just out for the money, they weren't just out for themselves, they weren't just out to overpower whoever they could overpower. And it was only after I met these guys—who were just, to me, really normal people who happened to be sur-

geons—that I said, "I can do this. I don't have to be like that to be a surgeon."

During the first two days I spent with Dr. Stephen, the tale of her experiences began to emerge. It was a terrible story, verging on the Kafkaesque. She showed me letters that supported and outlined pieces of it, and it certainly did add up to an attempt at "systematic annihilation." It occurred to me that she'd probably invited me to visit her just so I could hear the story and bear witness to it. It was like other stories of sexism and harassment that I'd heard from other women surgeons, but far worse, as if in her case the ugliness and evil ("evil" is not too strong a word) had been distilled. In this situation, I was faced with what historian Valerie Matsumoto calls "the force of the need to tell" (1996: 163). Kath Stephen needed a listener who would understand the implications of what had occurred. Later, when I recounted some of these experiences to other women surgeons and they elicited corresponding incidents that these women had not mentioned to me before, I realized that I needed to hear this story as much as Dr. Stephen needed to tell it. It is surely a worst-case scenario, but I suspect elements of it are familiar to many women surgeons.

Even before she was accepted into the surgical training program, Kath Stephen knew that some surgeons liked to create difficulties for women who wished to enter surgery.

When I was pregnant with my first child and I was a third-year medical student, we did a surgery rotation—there's a mandatory surgical rotation . . . I did the best I could to switch things around, but . . . It may have occurred during those first two weeks of the surgery rotation . . . I was told that if I didn't attend the first-day orientation where they taught you how to scrub, my letters recommending me for surgery residency would be guaranteed not to go out on time. And I ended up delivering on a Friday, and the first day of the surgery rotation was either a

Monday or Tuesday—I think it was a Tuesday. So I showed up for the orientation, which was stupid, because here I was, having been a nurse, having worked in the operating room for seven years already—I *knew* how to scrub. [She laughed.] This was not something I needed to be there for . . . And my milk had come in that day. I was in tremendous pain, and I just felt awful.

Kath Stephen then took two weeks off (which she had made up earlier in the year, ensuring that she would complete the full surgery rotation). The following year, she observed an incident involving the same senior surgeon:

During the fourth year, [I had] a male friend . . . whose wife was pregnant, and he was going through *his* surgery rotation. It was known that he was going into internal medicine, and the same surgeon who was the head of the medical students rotating through surgery—[my friend] asked [him] for a week off because his wife was pregnant. She was in her third trimester and having an uncomplicated pregnancy, but she was tired and wanted him home. And he [the senior surgeon] told him he could have a week off. "Just take it—we don't need you here . . . You're better off home anyway."

To a macho male surgeon, pregnancy and childbearing designate a body as being that of a vulnerable patient or wife, deserving of sympathy. There is, however, something intensely, unspeakably *wrong* about the body of a pregnant woman who claims to be a surgeon—that is, *in*vulnerable. Such a body must be punished for its presumption.

*Beginnings.* In her third year of medical school, Kath Stephen interviewed for residencies in both anesthesia and a surgical specialty. Although surgery was her first choice, she was worried that she might not be accepted into a surgical program. Since the surgical specialty was an "early match" (students who had chosen surgery were matched with a program before those who had chosen anesthesia), she would receive word on her acceptance or rejection before she had to sign up for an anesthesia list.[4] The surgery program in the Deep South was last on her list:

> Just because it was the Deep South, and I knew the culture was different. My interview with Dr. Allen [the divisional chief, an older surgeon near retirement] was very strange. [She laughed.] He wanted you to be the little—the sweet little nothing, and so I spent the night awake thinking whether I should put them on my list or not, because if you don't put them on your list, what if no one else wants you? Then you lose [the surgical specialty]. If you put them on your list and no one else wants you and you end up with them . . . [She laughed.] So I decided that I really wanted to be in surgery and put them on my list. And I did match there.

After Kath Stephen had "matched" there (they selected her; she selected them; she was assigned to the program), she discovered she was pregnant with her second child. At this time, she had to list the institutions where she wanted to do her internship (her first year of training). She did not want to intern at the Southern program, where trainees were on call every other night—she was scheduled to give birth just before she began—so she chose a program where she would work every third night. According to the written rules, a candidate could intern at one institution and do a residency at another. But when Dr. Allen learned that she wanted to do her first year elsewhere, he was incensed:

> He went into a rage. I was doing a third-year rotation in emergency medicine at an outlying hospital. He called me seven times collect that night to the emergency room. Got me out of my rotation to . . . *lambaste* me on the phone about how I was not committed, how I was going to lose my [specialty] spot. If I didn't come down there for the internship, then nothing else

was going to work—I had to be committed. This was the only way I could prove I was committed, was doing my internship there. And if I was going to give them this kind of problem, he wasn't going to—I could just forget the whole thing. [Dr. Allen did not yet know that she was pregnant.] And I wasn't going to tell him until I was . . . locked in place, [until] I had a surgery spot in [the specialty]. And so I said, "Yes, sir—anything you want, sir." I didn't realize this was going to cause such a commotion—I just thought it would be in my best interest. But I can see that I need to be, you know, "I'll be happy to do my internship [here]."

Once she had the place secured, Kath Stephen informed Dr. Allen and the senior surgeon in charge of the residency program that she was pregnant. Although they offered her three months off, she said she would take the minimum time off and be there as soon as possible to begin her internship.

The day after she graduated from medical school, Dr. Stephen and her husband moved to the Deep South, with their household goods loaded into a U-Haul. She was nine months pregnant. She gave birth nine days after the move, and started the surgery internship five weeks later. She entered the program three weeks late and managed, despite the fact that she had a newborn and a one-year-old at home, to work every other night, like her colleagues.[5]

*"I Had a Wonderful Time."* Dr. Stephen loved being a junior resident. "It was great!" she exclaimed. The men ignored her— but then, "they were all Southern boys" and did not know what to make of her. She was the only woman, and the first Northerner, in the specialty training program.[6]

While doing a rotation at another hospital, she found a mentor, Dr. Bates, who had been raised and trained in the North. "We were on extremely good terms together. We laughed. It was just a *wonderful* rotation—just wonderful. We just clicked." She enjoyed his subspecialty, and Dr. Bates encouraged her to go into it.

At the same time, she found that she loved research. She had conducted a few case studies in medical school, and Dr. Bates gave her a large project to organize. He set it up, and she did the actual work—designing the project, working with the statistician, corresponding with nurses in a number of hospitals to collect the data, and writing the paper, which Bates then edited. At this time, relations between the two were warm: they saw each other daily, and Dr. Bates began to discuss plans for her to enter his subspecialty and eventually become his partner.

> He wanted me to go into [his subspecialty] so badly that he paid for me to go up to Chicago and interview [for a fellowship]. He planned our future together as partners at the [hospital where he was based]—what he would do, what I would do, . . . how his interest would be this and my interest would be that, and how my going to Chicago would perfectly complement his fellowship in Los Angeles. He told me what he made. He told me what his benefits were . . . And he just—he had it all laid out for me as though he had his arm around me and I were his partner or sidekick.

Dr. Stephen was flattered and tempted, but eventually realized that the reason she was interested was not the subspecialty itself, but the fact that she liked Dr. Bates. There were other specializations she found more challenging: "It wasn't enough cutting and sewing for me." The following year she told him so. By this time, she was involved in other research projects with him. "Not realizing that this would upset him, or not acknowledging that it would, I assumed that just being straightforward and telling him—that he would understand and still support me in whatever decision I wanted to make in my academic career. Wrong!" Before writing a letter recommending her for a prestigious fellowship in another subspecialty, he insisted that Dr. Stephen withdraw her application to the area he had wanted her to enter. She did, and he then wrote the recommendation she had requested. Once he learned that she was not going to be his protégée and partner, however, he gradually withdrew his interest and support.

*Swan among the Ducklings.* It was clear to everyone that Dr. Stephen was a deviant in the department. She was not only a woman and a Northerner; she was also incredibly enthusiastic and industrious, and worked circles around the men.

> During my research rotation, I did more research than any other resident has ever done in the history of that program . . . So here I was, heavily into research. I was winning every award I applied for. I had one, two, three, four, eight poster presentations,[7] two invited seminars—no, wait: four poster presentations, eight oral presentations, seven of which were done with the residency, two invited seminars, and six publications, as a junior resident . . . And this is a slow, sleepy town . . . and a very clinical program. Okay? Well, being like that got me in trouble.

Unable to muster interest and support within her own department—with the exception of Dr. Bates, whose support began to wane when she announced she was not going into his subspecialty—she worked on research projects in other departments. At the same time, she was performing more operations than the men: "I worked hard to operate. I went to other departments and operated with other departments . . . ophthalmology, the division of plastics [plastic surgery] . . . I also was the first one to utilize the minor OR . . . [The other residents] might have done a few cases there, but since I was a nurse-anesthetist I was able to give these people sedation. I could do *lots* of things under local [anesthesia] which the other guys were not comfortable [doing]."[8] Naturally, showing up one's counterparts is not the way to win popularity contests, yet Dr. Stephen seems to have been unaware of how her activities affected the other residents. Every year, for example, the residents were supposed to submit the number of cases they had operated on, and these were then listed for accreditation.

> I was accurate in counting them up and I submitted them, and I had two hundred more cases than the senior residents. And the secretary told me that I had too many cases—she couldn't submit it like that. And did I really have these cases? "You know, you have to have op[erative] notes to back these up." I said, "Yes, I do [have operative notes]—that's not a problem." [But] she took it upon herself to just change the number of cases that I had, so that it was more in line with the seniors.' [Her voice became sarcastic.] I *couldn't* have [had] as many as the seniors, because I wasn't a senior.

I suspect that the secretary did not "take it upon herself"; she probably conferred, however indirectly, with senior surgeons before revising the figures. If her narrative is any indication, however, Dr. Stephen seems to have been oblivious to warning signs. She followed the overt rules for achievement, ignoring the covert social rules that govern people's behavior in various settings.

Of course, she was in the wrong program, in the wrong part of the country. In a hotshot Northern program, with young people as energetic and competitive as she, Dr. Stephen's enterprise might have been admired and rewarded—even coming from a woman. Dr. Bates, she said, had compared her to a racehorse: "Kathy, you are the racehorse. You are the racehorse. You are so far out in front of these other guys that you can't even see how far behind they are!" Yes, but a racehorse among the cart-horses resembles the swan among the ducklings in

Hans Christian Andersen's story. The one who is different from the rest of the group will be perceived as deformed, and the others will do their utmost to destroy the anomaly. Dr. Stephen expressed the same idea in different words: "This is the South," she said. "The nail that sticks out is going to be hammered in."

*"The Beginning of the End."* Gradually, Dr. Stephen became aware of ominous signs. Dr. Bates became less and less available. He kept encouraging her to continue their joint research, but was never there to discuss the details or to edit the papers she wrote about the findings. At one point, when she was already scheduled to present the results of their first joint study at a meeting in Bermuda, she received an invitation for the same day: she was being asked to come to Tucson, Arizona, to present her work on a nerve study conducted jointly with the departments of biochemistry and plastic surgery. She was not sure how to proceed. She asked Dr. Bates if he would present their joint paper, but he did not respond. A senior plastic surgeon arranged to have her presentation on the nerve study postponed by one day, so she made plans to go to Bermuda and then to Tucson. Two days before she was scheduled to leave, Dr. Bates told her by telephone that he would deliver the lecture and she would present a poster session, scheduled for a different hour. He then hung up, allowing no time for discussion. This last-minute change upset her travel schedule, and she had to change her flight reservations. The other residents were going to Bermuda and back, but she had to fly to Bermuda and then to Tucson and back, which was more expensive, especially with the last-minute change. "So I ended up doing it all. I went to Bermuda; I went to Tucson; I presented the work. And that was the beginning of the end. Well, not the *beginning* of the end—I guess it's well into it."

Dr. Stephen was in her fourth year. In April, the residents took their yearly in-service exams, where each was ranked on a percentile basis, compared with residents all over the country. In May, she attended the meetings in Bermuda and Tucson. Also in May, she went to another meeting where she and Dr. Bates had been invited to present their research results. Dr. Bates did not attend. During this meeting, one of Dr. Bates's mentors pulled her aside and asked, "Why are you doing this?"

> Not concerning the study, but concerning the whole thing. Because I was giving Bates all the credit during this meeting. "Dr. Bates did this and Dr. Bates did that, and da ta da ta da." He said, "Why are you doing this?" . . . He goes, "You're not getting paid for it." I said, "No."[9] I said, "Well, you know, Dr. Bates is my mentor, and he told me that I'd be first author." He said, "He's using you." And this was an older guy—I mean, he . . . must have been near seventy—and a big name. And all I could think of was, "Why is he saying that about one of his protégés? What an awful thing to say!" But he was right, and I should have seen it.

*Storm Clouds.*   At this stage, even Dr. Stephen, who had been oblivious to signs of trouble, was beginning to realize that she was in difficulties. In June, the residents received their scores on the in-service exams. She did not do particularly well; not abysmally, but not well. She had been spending too much time on research and not enough on reading.[10] As a result of that test, ten of the twelve residents, including Dr. Stephen, received a letter putting them on probation. At the same time, she received a letter from Dr. Bates directing her to submit in full, with photographs, and within the next ten days, all the research papers she had written with him.[11] Since he had spent eight months editing one paper, which he had not yet returned, she wrote back saying that she would send him the rest of the work, and that if she did not hear from him within a certain period of time, she would submit the finished paper for publication. He did not return the manuscript, and she did submit it to a surgical journal for publication. (It was accepted.) During the same month that she was put on probation and received the letter from Dr. Bates, she was asked to write a letter documenting how the travel funds for the trip to Bermuda and Tucson had been spent. (She later learned that the senior surgeons thought her airfare had been excessive and blamed her for appropriating money.) She sent the letter documenting the travel expenses. Later, she felt that the conjunction of these events—being put on probation, being pressured by Dr. Bates, and being questioned about the travel funds—was not accidental: they were part of an orchestrated attack.

In June, just before Dr. Stephen began her stint as chief resident, Dr. Bates called her to his office.

He was enraged. He closed the door, he stood up, he pounded his fists on the table, and he said, "Who do you think you are? You've been manipulative the whole time you've been in this program. I've just seen it now. You've tried to ruin this program by getting pregnant." I cut him off and said, "I only took three weeks off. I said I'd pay it back. *You're* the one that told me I didn't have to" . . . And he started coming at me with these things, how awful a person I was. And I said, "Look, if you're going to accuse me of all these things, are you going to accuse me of all these things at once and then let me rebut them all at the end? Or do you want to do it one by one? You tell me one thing and I'll rebut back." . . . And every time he'd say something, I'd rebut him. I'd say, "No, that's not the way it was. It was like this." And he'd say something else and I'd say, "No that's not the way it was. *You're* the one who told me to go there." . . . "No, that wasn't the way it was. *You're* the one that told me to present that the same day as this such and such." And he was just—he was just shaken. But very mad, very mad. And I walked out. With weak knees. But not having broken down and not having cried, which was very important to me. And not having really denigrated him . . . I never knowingly hurt his pride, which I felt was important.

It was obvious that Kath Stephen no longer had a mentor and protector.

*Assault.* On July 1, Dr. Stephen began her year as chief resident, on a rotation with Jack Curtin, the youngest of the four senior attending surgeons in the department. Dr. Curtin was a macho surgeon who favored the male residents, teaching them procedures that he did not allow her to perform. "When I was at the operating table with Jack Curtin, not a word would be said except, 'That's wrong!' 'Not there!' 'Not like that!' And yet when I eavesdropped without him knowing I was in the room, when he was teaching the guys, it would be, 'Okay, the vagus nerve is right here—yeah, that's right, good, good, okay, a little more of that, yeah, that's good. Now what's under there? Come on. All right."

At the end of July, she was paged in the operating room and told to go to the office of the divisional chief (who supervised her specialty department).

You never get paged out of the operating room to see the boss. I was frantic that something had happened to my children. I went to see [the chief], and he gave me a letter saying that I had two weeks to completely change or I'd be out of the program. And in that two weeks he expected me to do some things: I had to go see a psychiatrist; I had to have a physical exam; I had to document to him, with letters from every researcher I was working with, that I had completely severed research ties with them and was not working on any more research projects; and I had to increase my performance on the in-service exam at the end of the year, he said, "in line with the other residents in my program." (Now, one of these guys always got in the nineties [ninetieth percentile], you know.) Or I'd be out. I was just starting a forty-eight-hour solid call period, so I couldn't leave to go home—I couldn't leave to see anyone. My husband was out of town. I had no way of contacting him. He was gone.

She spent the forty-eight hours at the hospital completing her research commitments, and then went home. "I was immobile. I couldn't eat. I couldn't think. I couldn't talk. My two children and my mother-in-law [were there]. I just said, 'Could you stay with me? Could you just stay with me? Because I just don't know if I can do anything.' So she stayed with me, with the kids. Took care of the kids, while I basically just sat there." She then went to see a psychiatrist, who was affiliated with the medical school.

> He said, "You're not the first one I've seen from the department—there seem to be a lot of you flowing this way recently." And his eyes—getting wider, big as pies—looked at me. He sat next to me, straight across from me, looked me straight in the face, and said, "You haven't done anything wrong. Have you seen a lawyer?" And seeing a lawyer hadn't occurred to me— Rafe had thought of that. [The minute her husband had returned and had learned about the situation, he had located a lawyer.] And I said, "No." He goes, "Go see a lawyer." Now I had to go see a lawyer. [She laughed, near tears.]

In fact, Rafe had contacted a lawyer as soon as he'd returned to town and heard what had happened. Dr. Stephen then went to see this person—a woman who had at one time been a civil rights lawyer:

> I just was overflowing all over. I couldn't—I just was almost talking nonsense. And nothing made sense to me. I went and saw her, and I just spilled my guts, not knowing what I was talking about, and she looked at me and she said, "I know what

you have to say is important, but right now you just shut up and listen to me." She told me that I had to respond to the letter—that I should write the letter in my own words, bring it back to her, she would go over it. And from now on I just wasn't to talk . . . She also said, "I want you to see a different psychiatrist. I like the guy you're seeing—he's real good—but I want you to see a female psychiatrist, who has been through the [medical school training] program and came very close to suing them . . . If it comes to court, she will be more help to you, because I have seen the other psychiatrist on the stand and . . . I don't think he will do for you what she can do." So [she laughed], now I'm seeing *two* psychiatrists. Finally I stopped seeing the guy . . . I was just a *shambles*. I don't know how I went day to day. I went home. I slept all the time. I couldn't, you know, I couldn't—I couldn't function.

The second psychiatrist, who had been trained at the same university hospital, helped her rally her spirits.

"You're so depressed," she goes. "I can't believe what you're saying—nothing's changed in forty years." . . . So she put me on Prozac, which snapped me out of it in three weeks. And I was able to do what I needed to do. I was able to think, I was able not to worry, I was able to forget about everything else except studying for that test and smiling at Jack Curtin [who was supervising her and who disliked her] . . . I knew things were going on behind my back. Dr. Allen was telling residents to go and watch me and then come back and tell him how I was doing. Every day! The junior residents were told to come and *watch* me and see how I was doing. And see if I was anxious and see if I was stressed and see if I was irritable! And if I was irritable or not friendly—not friendly to the patients—then they were to go back and tell him.

The lawyer had told Dr. Stephen she should take the letter from the chief very seriously, because the senior surgeons were trying to expel her on the charge that she was not being a good doctor—a charge that would be difficult for them to prove. They could not expel her on the grounds that she was clinically or academically inept, which meant that they had to claim she was not being a good doctor and was unfriendly to patients. According to the lawyer, she needed to solicit support—verbally first, and then if possible in the form of letters. She managed to get verbal support from the other residents. "I talked to each one of them individually and asked them if they thought I should graduate the program or not. If anything I had done to them or that they had heard about—[would] they please ask me about it so that I could tell them. And did they think that I could be bad enough not to graduate the program. And every single one of them gave me a supportive response verbally—[but] I didn't have the guts to ask them to back it up on paper."

She then went to the nurses with a question-and-answer sheet: "Do you think Dr. Stephen is a good doctor? Do you think Dr. Stephen takes good care of her patients? Have you ever had a complaint from a patient about Dr. Stephen?" After each question, she had left a blank space where the nurses could insert their own comments, and at the bottom was a place for the nurse to sign her name. Dr. Stephen took this questionnaire to the nursing floors and, requesting permission from the head nurse, explained the situation to the nurses: "They thought this was a horrible thing to happen to me. Here I had been a nurse, I had come through the ranks—they were just *not* gonna let me crash. And I [got] a hundred letters from nurses." She also obtained letters from anesthesiologists and operating-room staff. OR personnel were so enthusiastic about the project that they photocopied the forms and left them all over the OR lounge, where Dr. Allen found one.

At this time, Dr. Stephen was having regular weekly meetings with Dr. Allen. His behavior was aggressive and unfriendly. He would stand while she sat—in fact, he would loom over her with his arms on the table, in what I would consider a highly intimidating stance (Dr. Stephen demonstrated for me). At one meeting, the chief confronted her with the form letter, demanding that she give him all the signed copies she had received. In his view, "they weren't mine," Dr. Stephen said. "They weren't worth anything anyway because they were solicited, and he should have them. They were his. And it took all the courage I had to say, 'No, sir—I cannot do that. I cannot give you those letters.' He wanted to know how many I had, and I wouldn't tell him. I remember he sat back and he looked up, and he goes, 'Why, there could be hundreds!' And as straightfaced as I could, I did not let on how many there were."

Dr. Stephen was convinced that the weekly meetings were an attempt to intimidate her—to "get me to take blame and shoot myself in the foot. They were tape recorded. Dr. Allen had a history of tape-recording sessions with residents [who had all been warned of this habit] . . . And he wasn't very adept at it. He'd fumble with the buttons. He'd turn the volume up and down. He'd ask you to say things louder, and when you started talking about a topic that he didn't want you to talk about, he'd tell you you couldn't talk about it. So you knew he was tape-recording you." At another weekly meeting, the chief threw her file down on the desk and said, "There's nothing in here!" "And when I told the lawyer this, she just laughed. She said, 'That's great!' I had . . . stuffed my file through the years with awards—I mean, any award I got, I sent a copy to [the chief's secretary] to put in the file. And letters from patients, and great clinical evaluations. And for him to throw it down on the desk and say, 'There's nothing in here' meant 'There's nothing in here that we can can [dismiss] you with.'"

Meanwhile, there were incidents—many of them orchestrated by Jack Curtin—which Dr. Stephen felt were designed to discredit her. But after four months on Dr. Curtin's service, she moved to another service and was then able to keep a low profile. I asked her if the attendings had tormented her all year. "Well, Dr. Curtin did. Toward the middle of the year, after about three or four months, Dr. Bates kind of wasn't a player anymore . . . I had gone underground. I wasn't making waves—I was staying out of everyone's way. Once I got off Jack Curtin's service, I could just—I could be an ostrich, I could be a hermit, I could show up for conference ten seconds before it started, leave ten seconds afterwards, and not say a word to anyone. And that's what I did."

Dr. Stephen needed a quiet, child-free place to study for the crucial in-service exams at the end of the year. "I had nowhere to go. I felt I couldn't study in the office; I couldn't study in the library; I couldn't even study in the hospital—that was such an unwelcoming place to me. All those places, I was unwelcome . . . So I got a little apartment, a little two-room apartment, put a card table and a folding chair and a coffeepot in there. It was a couple of blocks from the hospital, so I could actually go there if I had any time during the day, or whatever. I wasn't doing any research, so I went there and I studied well."

During this time, coached by the lawyer, Dr. Stephen sent several letters to the chief, putting the onus on the Division of Surgery to notify her if there were any problems with her performance.

> What they tried to do to me was to give *me* the responsibility for any problems. If there was a problem, *I* was the one who was supposed to come to *him*. And what [the lawyer] did was, she turned it around: if there was any problem, *he* was the one who was supposed to come to *me* . . . It documented—after it got turned around—that if Dr. Allen heard anything bad about me,

he was to call me immediately, and we would discuss it . . . A month later we sent him a letter—I sent him a letter—saying, "I'm so glad to know that there have been no problems since blah, blah, blah." Okay . . . Then things kind of let up.

Following the lawyer's advice, Dr. Stephen never let the senior surgeons know directly that a lawyer was involved; she left them guessing. After about eight weeks of meetings with the chief, the scheduled meetings started tapering off. In April she took the in-service exams, and in June learned the results: she had gotten the highest score in the residency program (ninetieth percentile). But she was still on probation. Since she could not graduate while on probation, and thought the fact that she had not formally graduated might come back to haunt her, she solicited a letter that would take her off probation. It had been announced that Dr. Allen, the chief, was retiring the following month, and so she asked Dr. Bates, who was head of the residency program, to write the letter (which had to be co-signed by Allen). He did so; but rather than acknowledging that she had gotten the best in-service score in the department (in the ninetieth percentile), his letter announced that she had scored 76 percent—which was correct, but not the relevant number.[12]

"So you got out?" I asked. "So I got out," she replied.

I was denied my senior-class trip, which the other residents took, paid for by the department. I was not allowed to take any trips that last year. [They said that] I needed the time to study. An abstract that I had already submitted [I was told] to retract, which I did. The [research] paper with Dr. Bates was delayed, and two years later he changed the listing of authors, so that he was the first author and I was the second author . . . And the other two residents got to leave a week early, [but] I had to stick it out to the last day. It was the standard for the chief residents to be able to leave at least a few days early. But I had to stay until the very last day.[13]

She then commuted for a year to a Northern city, where she did a fellowship with a world-famous surgeon in the subspecialty she was most interested in; she was one of only seven women who had held this fellowship. She learned that during her final year of training, a senior surgeon in the division had written to this surgeon, asking him to withdraw his fellowship offer. He had responded that the offer was in writing and he could not withdraw it.

Dr. Stephen said that although the surgery program has terminated quite a few women, and has threatened to terminate others, such as herself, she knows of no instances when they terminated a male resident. One man, who was technically inept, was channeled into another specialty. Another was arrogant and unpleasant and thought he knew everything; the nurses hated him. He once killed a child by inserting a catheter backward into its heart. In the subsequent lawsuit, the attending surgeon was not sued—only the resident and the hospital were deemed liable. The family won the suit, since the nurses had documented what had happened. Yet after all this, the resident was not terminated; he was encouraged to enter radiology in another state.

*In Retrospect.* Dr. Stephen later realized—and admitted to me—that she had made serious mistakes during her training. Ruefully, she quoted a publication issued by the Association of Women Surgeons for the benefit of residents: "Your aim is not to do research or anything else; your aim is to get through the program." "I wish I had had that at the time," she said. Intellectually and surgically gifted, she was apparently socially and politically blind. Obviously she needed a mentor, to advise her about the best course and to caution her against some of the mistakes she was making (such as spending too much time on research and not enough on keeping up with the literature;

failing to make friends with her counterparts; neglecting to win a wider base of support among senior surgeons).

As for Dr. Bates, his own mentor seems to have been right: he was using Dr. Stephen. He coopted her imagination, energy, and drive, but discarded her as soon as it became clear that he could not profit from them indefinitely. He bet on the "race-horse" only so long as it was in his stable. He did not advise her on how best to get through the program—how *not* to make enemies. She was fine so long as he ran interference for her, but he stopped protecting her when it no longer benefited him. Her welfare does not seem to have concerned him; per-haps he did not see it as separate from his own. Once her welfare *was* clearly separated from his, he lost interest.

Dr. Stephen was obviously the wrong body in the wrong place, in a geographic area where women's bodies had specific movements, meanings, and symbolic values that were alien to her. Not only her gender but everything about her habitus was wrong: she was the first *Northerner*, male or female, in the train-ing program. The three women who had previously managed to finish the program had all been Southerners: wrong gender but a familiar habitus.

One evening, while I was staying at Dr. Stephen's home, she received a visit from her friend Dr. Albright—a chunky, confident, competent-looking hand surgeon. Dr. Albright said she had been raised on a farm in the region, had financed her medical education by doing construction work during the summer, and had done a fellowship at the university hospital where Dr. Stephen had been trained. She related an anecdote about her fellowship year. Seated in the doctor's lounge read-ing a magazine, she'd been asked by a senior surgeon: "What are you reading, recipes?" "The only recipe I know is for Sakrete," she'd replied, referring to a brand of concrete. Dr. Albright had been communicating embodied information, as well as a veiled warning: anyone who can mix and use concrete has the right body for a surgeon. At the same time, she had been imparting additional information about bodily and social space: I am not a southern lady, but my *habitus* is familiar. I'm a Southern countrywoman, capable of physical feats that effete city folk, male and female, cannot match. So don't mess with me, buster!

If Dr. Stephen had been a Southern lady or countrywoman, if her habitus had been familiar to the men who trained her, perhaps she would have made it through the program with less difficulty. Perhaps not. It is quite possible that Pat Hakimian, the "bitch" she was warned against, was Southern. Misogyny is an equal-opportunity destroyer. Dr. Stephen, however, had more than three strikes against her: the wrong gender; the wrong female habitus; a mentor who turned against her; and a lack of senior women surgeons to provide embodied tutelage. In retrospect, it is remarkable that she finished the program. Without the aid of a woman lawyer and a psychiatrist, she may not have succeeded. As it is, the emotional price was disastrously high.

# SURGEONS IN THIS DAY AND AGE

What can Dr. Stephen's terrible tale tell us—besides exposing us to a kind of viciousness that we might prefer not to know about? To say that there is a double standard in male-dominated fields is accurate, but almost a platitude. We can note that a woman in such a malevolent environment is in a double bind: if she is *not* exceptional, she'll probably not be good enough to make it through; if she *is* exceptional, she'll be the nail that sticks out and gets hammered in. But that too, if not quite a platitude, brings little light to the issues involved. The most illuminating analysis of such misogyny is, again, provided by Bourdieu: "The ultimate values, as they are called, are never anything other than the primary primitive dispositions of the body, 'visceral' tastes and distastes, in which the group's most vital interests are embedded . . . The sense of distinction, the *discretio* (discrimination) which demands that certain things be brought together and others kept apart, . . . responds with visceral, murderous horror, absolute disgust, metaphysical fury, to everything which . . . passes understanding, that is, the embodied taxonomy, which, by challenging the principles of the incarnate social order, especially the socially constituted principles of the sexual division of labour and the division of sexual labour, violates the mental order, scandalously flouting common sense" (1984: 474–475).

Dr. Stephen never forgot that on her first day in the training program, someone she did not even know warned her to stay away from another woman resident, described as a "bitch." Suppose that Kath Stephen, the bitch-to-be, and Pat Hakimian, the bitch, had joined forces? And then made common cause with the other six women who were eventually forced to leave the program? Were the women too powerless to lend any strength and support to one another? Would the stigmatized position of each rub off on the others? Or could they have shared notes, strategies, and suggestions for counselors in the hospital or medical school—and, if necessary, lawyers' addresses—and learned from one another's predicaments? I don't know the answer. I have not survived a surgical training program (and lack the iron to do so), nor am I familiar with the Southern milieu.[1]

Ben Franklin's advice during the American Revolution is apposite: we must hang together, or we will all hang separately. In unity, there is not necessarily strength; but in division, there is surely weakness.

The Association of Women Surgeons publishes a pamphlet, "The Pocket Mentor," that warns against many of the mistakes Dr. Stephen made. It discusses relevant issues, from politics to pregnancy to gender discrimination. The association also has a list of mentors—women surgeons who can be contacted for advice on various issues: contract disputes, harassment, isolation, residency. If Dr. Stephen had had access to such women during her training, she might have sidestepped some of the problems she encountered, or benefited from informed, sympathetic advice in dealing with them. Even more illuminating would have been the day-by-day opportunity to "learn by body" from another woman, as her male peers did from men.

("Okay, the vagus nerve is right here—yeah, that's right, good, good, okay, a little more of that, yeah, that's good. Now what's under there? Come on. All right.")[2] As she incorporated surgical techniques, she would also have been absorbing embodied knowledge of how to be a woman surgeon—how to conduct herself and survive in the face of the machismo and misogyny her peers were undoubtedly assimilating from senior staff members such as Jack Curtin.

Many of the women surgeons I studied preferred not to think of themselves as women—as *women* surgeons. They were surgeons, pure and simple, who just happened to be women. They did not join women's organizations, such as the Association of Women Surgeons, because they did not define themselves *primarily* as women, nor did they want to be so defined by others.[3] I suspect this is how neurosurgeon Frances Conley perceived herself for much of her career: as "one of the guys."[4] I doubt, however, that the guys ever perceived Conley as one of the guys. Conley learned that she had to think of herself as a woman, as well as a surgeon, since that is how she was thought of by everyone else, and she became what I think of as a "born-again feminist." Today, she lectures and writes about sexual discrimination and the need for women to join together.[5] Alas, a woman surgeon who thinks of herself as "one of the guys" shows a tragicomic resemblance to Winnie-the-Pooh holding on to a balloon and floating up into the sky, asking hopefully if he does not resemble a black cloud. No, you look like a bear with a balloon, Pooh is told.

A woman surgeon has little choice. She is a woman as well as a surgeon—that cannot be changed. She has a woman's body, a woman's movements, a lifetime of experiences as a woman. She can perceive herself as one of the guys; she can epitomize the mystique of the iron surgeon; she can be more macho than the men, defining caring and compassion as the subjective, unscientific, touchy-feely province of nurses and social workers. Nevertheless, she will always be a macho *woman*, with a different habitus from that of a macho man— just as the fatherly habitus of a compassionate man differs from the motherly habitus of a compassionate woman. Seniors, colleagues, patients, and nurses will react to her as a woman (not as a neutral category—not as one of the guys—but as a woman).

Perhaps someday this difference will be less significant and will no longer elicit double standards, double binds, discrimination, and harassment. Perhaps someday a woman's body will be welcomed as subject *and* object in death-haunted vocations, as instrumental doer *and* passive done-to, as rescuing hero *and* she who is to be rescued. Until that day, a woman surgeon would do well to heed Ben Franklin's maxim.

## A CHANGING PROFESSION, AN UNCERTAIN FUTURE

In 1984 I asked a young surgeon whose compassionate manner I admired whether he would want his son to become a surgeon. He responded negatively. Patients had unreasonable expectations, he said—they assume that every problem can be taken care of and every procedure will turn out well. "It's no fun anymore," he declared, and a chief resident joining the conversation echoed his words: "It's no fun anymore" (Cassell 1991: 182–209). Of seventeen men who were asked if they would want their sons or daughters to become surgeons, thirteen replied that they would not.[6] The theme of "no fun" ran like a dark current through the surgeons' conversations. The phrase "this day and age" was a kind of shorthand for an upheaval in American medicine, particularly in surgery. The canons of practice, procedure, relationships, and reimbursement were all changing—to the surgeons' minds, for the worse. "It's not a good field anymore," said one man, describing how he had discouraged his three children from entering surgery. "You lack independence. You lack freedom."

These conversations took place more than a decade ago, and the changes have accelerated. Surgeons' fees, freedom, and working conditions are increasingly constrained. Their decisions are challenged and countermanded by faceless entities handing down edicts by telephone; on occasion, they are forced to lie to obtain the care they believe a particular patient requires.[7] Most galling for many is the diminution and devaluation of the surgeon's charisma. Heroes who display "manliness," "manhood," "manly courage" are no longer glorified as they once were; and surgeons are no longer considered heroes as they once were. Said one man:

> We're gonna be the first generation—my generation of physicians—who are *not* going to encourage their children to go into medicine . . . I always looked forward, like when I first started private practice, that [my partner] and I would be turning over the practice to his sons and my son and my daughter—you know, a family practice. But now, I don't know. Everybody's considering me a vendor, or I'm a provider. I'm a vendor, and this is a consumer. They took away the integrity! . . . No one trusts us. There's no integrity.

The charismatic surgical hero is being replaced by the "health care provider"—a petty bureaucrat, interchangeable with thousands of others, who treats patients as interchangeable cogs.[8]

The changes in medicine and surgery are wide-ranging, profound, and painful to many. Not only practices but perspectives—once believed integral to the profession—are shifting. Among these changes is an erosion of the mentor-student bond. Reverence for one's mentor has been a fundamental aspect of Western medicine from its earliest days.[9] The wording of the Hippocratic Oath—"To consider dear to me as my parents him who taught me this art; to live in common with him and if necessary to share my goods with him; to look upon his children as my own brothers; to teach them this art if they so desire without fee or written promise"—indicates that the filial relationship involves mentor as well as protégé. If the teacher is to be honored as a symbolic father, the student in turn is nurtured as a symbolic son.[10]

In this day and age the traditional structures of respect, obedience, and nurturance are breaking down under the pressures of what the sociologist Paul Starr terms "the coming of the corporation" (1982: 420). This disintegration is exquisitely painful to those who assume that such relationships are fundamental to the practice of medicine. Once, in 1996, I went with a woman-surgeon friend to dine at a crowded Chinese restaurant, and the two of us were ushered to a group table. The man sitting next to us turned out to be an oncologist who had trained at the same urban university hospital as my friend. He said that when he had finished his training, he and two colleagues had organized a group practice in a small suburban community. They had been so successful that they'd recently taken on a third partner. Then the hospital where he had trained announced that it was going to open a satellite cancer center in his community. "It doesn't matter who gives the best care," said the oncologist. "Patients will go to the famous name." The young doctor who had just entered their practice quit: "There's nothing for me here," he announced. The oncologist, seeing that the competition would kill his group practice, went to the man who had trained him: "How can you do this to me?" His former chief responded, "I'm not your father. This is business!" "I'm fifty-five years old," said the oncologist, "too young to retire. Where will I go? What will I do?"

The surgeon with whom I was dining had her own worries. The health maintenance organization she worked for—the oldest in the city and one of the oldest in the United States, which had cared for generations of teachers, police officers, and other city employees—was in trouble.[11] New for-profit HMOs were luring unions by offering chrome-plated deals and cut-rate prices, and she feared for her job. "I should have gone into law. Medicine is the wrong field to be in today," she said ruefully.

## WOULD YOU DO IT AGAIN?

Since I began studying surgeons in 1983, more and more women have been entering the profession. Between 1970 and 1993 the number of women in surgery increased tenfold, and it is still growing. How do these women evaluate their careers? Would they advise other women to go into surgery? Would they do it again? In my earliest tape-recorded interviews, I asked each surgeon what advice she would give to young women thinking of going into surgery. Later in my research I posed the question in two different ways, first asking what advice the surgeon would give, and then inquiring whether she would choose the same career if she could live her life over again.

Some of the women expressed distress at the developments of "this day and age"; the others, however, appeared delighted to be surgeons. The doubts were instructive. One woman who said she would do it again continued, "But I wasn't prepared for the politics, for all the forms I have to fill out, and the medical politics . . . I used to think I would do third-world surgery, and everyone told me that wasn't a good idea . . . If I had to do it over again, I think I might do third-world surgery. I might still even do it, one of these days." A woman in her first year of practice said doubtfully, "Well, I love what I do. But I don't know if I'd go into medicine again." "Wait ten years and then see how you feel," advised a male colleague. "In fifteen years, I'll be fifty-five and the kids will be educated and I'll retire. I have lots of things I'd like to do with my time," he declared, predicting that surgeons are all going to start retiring early.

Three women said that they would not become surgeons if they could make the choice again. They mentioned the changes in medicine and surgery, the curtailed autonomy, the diminished respect shown doctors. Said one, "I don't like being a physician in a time when there's such antiphysician sentiment. I don't like being concerned when someone asks me what I do, and they say, '*Oh!*' Even my brother: 'Oh, well, you're out to make a buck, like all of 'em.'" Another said, "In this day and age, because medicine is changing and therefore doctors are changing, you have to be a businessperson—you have to be more concerned about money now than ever before. Ten years ago, that wasn't the case. You went to medical school fairly cheaply, you paid off your loans within ten years, and you made a huge salary. Your wife didn't work and you still had a home with a tennis court and a pool, and your kids went to private schools. Now, it takes you thirty years to pay off your student loan." When I inquired how much she owed, she responded, "About $25,000, which is low." The third woman was even more disillusioned:

> You're in a constant state of aggravation, frustration, harassment. You're harassed by utilization people,[12] you're harassed by obnoxious patients, you're constantly feeling pressure from all kinds of extraneous bureaucrats and functionaries that have no business even *looking* at you, let alone telling you what to do or how you can do it. The practice of medicine isn't the practice of medicine any more . . . In private practice . . . you have to justify hospital admissions to some nurse-functionary on the

other end of the line, and you have to be very careful about your statistics—[careful] that you don't keep patients longer than what is the norm in the bell curve, because you're going to be dropped from the [hospital surgery] program.

Even worse than the things I've already mentioned is the relationship you have with patients—is that patients have no respect as a rule anymore for physicians. They walk into [your office] with this adversarial, confrontational air that I find *absolutely intolerable,* absolutely intolerable. I have no patience for people who walk in thinking they know more than I do, thinking that they are going to tell me what I am going to do for them and how I am going to do it. And . . . you encounter more and more of that type of patient.

Two women gave what seemed to me to be equivocal—or conflicted—responses when asked what advice they would offer a young woman thinking of going into surgery. Each had children, was married to a doctor, and took primary responsibility for home and children. Young women choosing surgery, said one, would really be "biting off an awful lot. Now, it could give them a wonderfully fulfilling life, and in a large part mine is, but . . . if one is not careful, you just give your self away, and you turn around and you think, 'What's left? Who's this? Is this really living, or is this just getting all the things done that need to be done and all the people in the right place? And is this really what I would consider, what I would choose, if I had X number of days left to experience?'" The other said: "I would advise anyone going into medicine now to think twice . . . Because it's just too hard. And especially [for] a woman, I think, it's too hard, and there are too many demands, and there are too many things that—whether you consciously decide to put them off or not do them—there are too many things that you have to give up. If you always wanted to do this and you never

thought anything else would make you happy, you're probably gonna have the dedication to make it palatable. [But] if in
the back of your mind there's always this other thing that you
thought you might have done, you're gonna wish you'd done
the other thing." When I inquired, "How about surgery as a
branch of medicine?" she replied: "Think even ten times
harder about doing that than doing some other branch of
medicine, because it's more demanding . . . Surgical residency
is more demanding than any other residency. My internship
was more demanding than [that of] any of my friends who
were interns in something else . . . My day always started earlier and lasted longer than [that of] somebody who was in a
nonsurgical field. I think it's a tough life."

Some women who said they would do it again specified that
surgical training, and possibly surgery itself, were not suitable
for a woman who wanted marriage and children. One surgeon
advised women entering the field to be single-minded: "You
have to have tunnel vision to do surgery. I don't think it's a life
for someone who wants to get married and have children,
although I know other women have done it." Said another: "A
year or two ago, [when] one of the cardiologists . . . said something about his daughter being a surgeon, I advised him
against it. I told him that it was swimming upstream." She said
she would caution *all* women thinking of entering surgery that
they would be going upstream. "If you don't mind, and you
thrive on the nontraditional and out-of-the-ordinary, and you
don't want what is traditionally wanted in this culture, then I
would say, 'Go for it!' . . . But if you have traditional wishes
and want it all, you won't get it all. You will not get it all."

Some thought that subspecialties might be more appropriate
than general surgery for a woman who wanted children. One
surgeon said, "I would encourage them very aggressively to

look at the pediatrics and dermatology of surgery—to look at areas of surgery that might allow them some control of their private life."

Interestingly, Kath Stephen—despite her bitter experiences during training—responded: "Well, I love what I do, and I think it's the right career for me. It is exactly the career for me. The road to get there [long pause] . . . Yes, I still would have done it."

Many women, however, expressed few doubts. "Yes, in a heartbeat!" responded one. "Absolutely! I can't imagine being anything but a surgeon," said another. A surgeon in her sixties, who had finished her training thirty-four years before, said: "I think it's a wonderful field. I think it's emotionally very rewarding and technically very rewarding, and it's a fun thing to do, and it's exquisitely interesting." Another, in her forties, observed: "You have to think of what you want to do every single day of your life . . . When I thought of surgery, I was always excited."

One young surgeon summed it up. As a medical student, she had been assigned to a resident who had once said something puzzling to her. Years later, seeing him at a surgical meeting, she asked him about it:

I said, "Cliff, I remember . . . back in the olden days, when I was a third-year medical student thinking about going into surgery, . . . your telling me that you only do this if you can't do anything else." And I said, "What do you mean, if you can't?" This was three o'clock in the morning and . . . we had come from the operating room and were going to the emergency room. And I said, "Oh, man!"—wide-eyed and excited and enthusiastic—"Oh, this is so cool!" And he said, "You only do this if you can't do anything else." And I remember saying to him, "Well, I'm a bright kid—I'm at the top of my class." (Thinking to myself, "I can do whatever I want to do.") And he said, "No, I don't mean that. I mean if you can't get up in the morning and face going to do something that requires less physical stamina and less hours and less grief, then you do this. [She laughed.] Because you can't face the day doing something else."

When I asked what advice she would give to young women thinking of going into surgery, she replied: "Do it, if you can't do anything else. That's what I would tell them."

/ / / / / / / / / / / / / / / / / / / / /

# NOTES

## 1. "What's an Anthropologist Doing Studying Surgeons?"

1. "I seem to gravitate to doing things that are difficult just because I crave challenge," wrote surgeon Rhonda Cornum in a letter from Persian Gulf region, where she was subsequently taken prisoner in the 1991 war. Cornum, a major in the U.S. Army, described how going into combat was "in some ways . . . a personal test to see if you have the 'right stuff'" (Cornum 1996: 12). This is the surgical temperament par excellence.

2. For example, Kleinman (1986, 1988, 1995); M. J. Good et al. (1992); B. Good (1994); Scheper-Hughes and Lock (1987); Lock and Gordon (1988); Martin (1987).

3. Moore is a British social anthropologist, Gatens an Australian philosopher; both are feminists. The work of Susan Bordo (1993), a feminist philosopher, has also been stimulating. Like myself, all three are interested in the consequences of inhabiting a *woman's* body rather than that of a man.

4. Emily Martin, for example, is concerned with "the complex ways scientific discoveries lead to new cultural understandings of life and personhood" (1992: xviii) and with differences in the way that physicians and women understand women's bodily processes. Many of the contributors in Thomas Csordas' edited volume (1994) are preoccupied with Foucauldian concepts, using their concepts and data to illustrate or attack Foucault's ideas. They are concerned (as Terence Turner's article states) with "theoretical, ontological and epistemo-

logical issues," wishing to contribute (as Csordas states in the front of the volume) "to a phenomenological theory of culture and self." I am doing something far simpler and less ambitious: attempting to understand and explain the phenomena I encountered when conducting fieldwork.

5. See Bordo (1993: 225).


## 2. Bodies of Difference

1. On the surgical embodiment of "manliness, manhood, manly courage," see Cassell (1986, 1987, 1991: 33–44); on firefighters, see Kaprow (1991); on fighter pilots, see Wolfe (1979). On race car drivers, a 1983 film, *Heart Like a Wheel* (Aurora, Charles Rovin), presents the story of a woman attempting to enter the phallicized world of auto racing.

2. The phallic element may be symbolic or overt. Thus, among the "games" that firemen play in their all-male firehouses, which Kaprow (1990) compares to Amazonian men's houses, are "scrotum on the head," and an unnamed diversion consisting of taking morning roll call naked, which involves sliding down the pole unclothed. The men have been legally enjoined from playing the second "game" when female firefighters are present, since this has been deemed "sexual harassment" (Kaprow n.d.).

3. Although I may be belaboring the obvious, let me point out the difference between "heroism" and (to invent a culturally impossible word) "heroine-ism." The OED definitions of "hero" and "heroine" are instructive. "Hero" is glossed as "1. A name given (as in Homer) to men of superhuman strength, courage, or ability, favored by the gods. 2. A man distinguished by extraordinary valor and martial achievements; one who does brave or noble deeds; an illustrious warrior." "Heroine" is defined as "1. In ancient mythology, a female intermediate between a woman and a goddess; a demigoddess. 2. A woman distinguished by exalted courage, fortitude, or noble achievements." The first thing one learns about a heroine is that she is a mythical creature; one then learns that although, like the hero, she possesses courage, unlike the hero—whose ability, strength, and valor are emphasized—she is defined by her "fortitude" and noble "achievements." One gets the impression that a heroine is characterized by her noble *soul;* a hero, by his noble *deeds.*

4. Murphy and Murphy (1974: 85–100); Gillison (1993: 265–276); Herdt (1981).

5. Adams analyzes the institution's rituals known as the "Ratline" and "Break Out," observing: "As I watched Break Out in 1993, the ritual seemed less of a 'bizarre ordeal' [as it was described by supporters] than a metaphorical birth, an impression which the [institution's] cadets corroborated when we analyzed the ritual later. I was further struck not by the intensity of 'hazing' but by the tenderness of the seniors, who are called 'dykes.' Why, at a school dedicated to heterosexual men, would its major ritual recall childbirth, and its central role, female homosexuality?" Adams' students at a nearby women's college compared these rituals to those described in the early literature on the male cults of Melanesia and Amazonia, where the men direct initiation rituals that achieve a symbolic rebirth, transforming boys into men; these peoples reason that women give birth to boys, but only *men* can give birth to men. Adams compares this to the antebellum slogan of the Southern military institution she studied: "Give us your boy and we'll send you a man."

6. Kaprow (n.d.) argues that this process is beginning to occur in firefighting. I believe it is further along in surgery.

7. Data for surgeons in private practice are difficult to find. Medical professors' salaries are comparable, however, if one includes "supplemental compensation"—that is, income generated by the surgeon, which may include bonuses, consultant fees, and a percentage of patient fees; in 1995–1996, these averaged from $241,500 a year for orthopedists to $433,400 a year for neurosurgeons (Smith 1996: 12). All over the country, however, as hospitals shrink and merge under pressure from managed care, senior doctors and nurses are being let go. The higher the salary, the more vulnerable the health care professional. A world-famous transplant surgeon was dismissed as a department head when two Harvard hospitals merged (*New York Times*, January 26, 1997: A1). Among the medical specialties, surgeons are the most highly remunerated, which may make them more susceptible to such cost-cutting. Because few women surgeons are full professors or department heads (whose salaries are even higher than professors'), they are less vulnerable to cost-cutting. Naturally, such cuts create a climate of fear among health care professionals.

8. The number of women surgeons grew from 485 in 1970 to 4754 in 1993 (Rogers 1995). The *proportion* of women in surgery increased

more slowly, from less than 1 percent in 1970 to 5 percent in 1993. In 1994, the proportion of women residents in surgical specialties was 13.9 percent (Sheldon 1996: 526; see also Kwakwa and Jonasson 1996).

9. In the early 1980s, an intern in the first hospital I studied (the only woman in the training program) had been accepted into a neurosurgery program, which she planned to enter after two years of general surgery training. The neurosurgery chief who had accepted her application, however, was replaced by another man who announced that he did not want a woman, and canceled her acceptance. He did not wish to meet her or know anything about her; the fact that she was a woman was enough to disqualify her. Unable to find a place in another neurosurgery program, she left surgery for radiology (despite the fact that the chief of general surgery had offered her a slot in his program). "All I ever wanted to be since I was a little girl was a brain surgeon," she lamented. She told me that, at that time, there were twenty-six senior women neurosurgeons in the United States.

10. This is pediatrician Perry Klass's description of the ways she changed during medical school (Klass 1987).

11. "The surgeon is seen as a John Wayne type," observed a woman surgeon (Kinder 1985: 103), who criticized this approach, suggesting that "qualities that women in general bring quite unselfconsciously to patient care and resident and student teaching," such as sensitivity, warmth, and compassion, might improve the way surgery is taught, learned, and practiced.

12. For an informed and thoughtful summary of issues and publications on women in medicine, see Lorber (1985). (Lorber 1984 offers a more extended discussion.) As to women surgeons, all I could locate at the time was one mail survey (Ramos and Feiner 1989) of 386 women surgeons. Since then, although I have come across a number of articles and publications in medical and surgical journals devoted to women in medicine and/or surgery, I still know of no other full-scale study of women surgeons. When, in 1995, I presented some of my findings at the annual meetings of Women in Neurosurgery, in San Francisco, and the Association of Women Surgeons, in New Orleans, none of the women mentioned additional research on women surgeons.

13. In 1993 I learned of the existence of the Association of Women Surgeons and promptly joined. This organization publishes a listing of

members, with addresses and phone numbers and, when their newsletter mentioned my research project, I received letters and phone calls from women surgeons all over the country offering to participate in the study. I noticed, however, that thirteen of the eighteen women surgeons I had already studied did *not* belong to this organization. Consequently, drawing my study population from the AWS (which I did not do) would have skewed my sample toward those women who identified themselves as *women* surgeons rather than primarily as *surgeons*, which is the way many of the women I studied spoke of, and apparently conceptualized, themselves.

14. I omitted obstetrician-gynecologists and ophthalmologists from my sample, however. Persuaded that they were a different population, I used the fact that these specialties had separate training programs to justify this decision.

    The American College of Surgeons and the Association of Women Surgeons, on the other hand, include obstetrician-gynecologists. Several seemed offended that I had ignored their specialty: they were "the same as" surgeons, they told me. Several surgeons, however, privately communicated their conviction that obstetrician-gynecologists were "different."

    A few medical schools are setting up separate orthopedic training programs. At the time I was planning and conducting research for this study, however, such programs were rare, and I thus included orthopedists.

15. Included with the letter were a curriculum vitae, to indicate I was not a novice, and reprints of published articles on surgeons, to show that my goal was to study rather than smear surgeons. Surgeons are all shielded by secretaries; it was necessary to send the material, inform each woman that I was going to telephone her, and then telephone three to six times in order to discuss the study with her and learn whether she would participate. One woman put me off for an entire year, another for nine months (their secretaries kept advising me to telephone again in three to six months), before both refused to participate in the study.

16. Many patients were in such difficult and painful circumstances that I did not wish to burden them with the details of my research; there were almost always other medical personnel present, so that I did not stand out. Surgeons varied in informing patients who I was. When anyone posed a direct question (such as "What kind of doctor

are you?"), I described my project. Every patient—and nurse, for that matter—who learned my identity seemed delighted that it was the *doctor* who was being observed.

17. I spent a week at a fourth site, as a houseguest of the surgeon I studied (see Chapter 8).

18. Naturally, this is a very (probably overly) broad generalization. Medical sociologists have a tradition of studying Western doctors; and ever since Arthur Kleinman, who is both an anthropologist and a physician, took over the chair of the Department of Social Medicine at Harvard, social scientific studies of "biomedicine" have increased. (See Hahn and Gaines 1985 for one of the earliest collections of anthropological essays, published in a series edited by Kleinman.) Moreover, in the past fifteen or twenty years, as grant money for travel has become scarcer and colonial administrations have been replaced by indigenous governments favoring indigenous researchers, a growing number of anthropologists have discovered the delights of studying their own society, a practice they formerly disdained.

19. Cassell (1987b, 1989); Wax and Cassell (1979); Cassell and Wax (1980); Cassell and Jacobs (1987).

20. At an anthropological meeting I became acquainted with Pearl Katz, who had studied surgeons; but at that time, she had published only one article on her researches (1981).

21. In all honor, I was unable to conceal the subject of my study, when asked. Questions of moral self-regulation, however, turned out to be the issues most concealed from me while I was conducting research, and although I learned enough to devote a few chapters to it, I ended by conducting a more traditional anthropological study of an exotic tribe.

22. A number of women would notice when I shivered in the OR, and would direct a nurse to obtain a jacket or blanket for me. Several went out of their way to instruct me in getting from Point A to Point B, when they learned that I had a defective sense of direction. An exhausted chief resident, who had been on call for thirty-six hours, participated in my tape-recorded interview conducted at her home, then left her husband and baby, got into her car, and led me to the highway. "Drive safely!" she called as we parted.

23. Charles Bosk quotes a surgeon who makes the same comment, refer-

ring to the need to teach, learn, and evaluate surgery in the operating room (1979: 13).

24. With the exception of psychoanalysis, which deals with the psyche (and was until comparatively recently an exclusively *medical* specialty only in the United States), Western medicine treats the bodies of patients, who are viewed as autonomous and distinct units (D. R. Gordon 1988b; E. J. Cassell 1991: 3–10). In contrast, non-Western therapies are more likely to treat the patient as a member of a social group; not only the body but the patient's relationships must be healed (e.g., Turner 1967; Finkler 1994; Kleinman 1995: 36–37).

25. "Feeling, touching, seeing, all have to be learned by the novice," notes D. R. Gordon (1988a: 274), quoting a surgeon's account of his first appendectomy (Nolen 1970: 48), when he put his hand into the patient's abdomen and was unable to identify what he felt (1988: 274).

26. I'm indebted to John Singleton (personal communication) for this concept.

27. This hierarchy, with surgeons at the peak and psychoanalysts on the lowest rung, is widely acknowledged in medicine. In recent years, many psychiatrists have abandoned the Freudian "talking cure" for a reliance on medications that affect bodily functions. Not surprisingly, such biologically based practitioners consider themselves superior to psychoanalytically based colleagues who are less involved with the body (Luhrmann 1994).

28. The rivalry between internists and surgeons is much discussed and the topic of a good deal of banter, but on occasion is quite real. Surgeons often do believe that internists tend to overintellectualize, while many internists are convinced that surgeons act without sufficient thought.

29. For a discussion of some of these issues, see Haraway (1991).

30. E.g., Wilson (1975, 1978); Moir (1991).

31. The biological-differences argument was used to bar women from higher education. "In Germany, the renowned Munich anatomist Theodor von Bischoff summed up a generation's thinking in 1872 when he argued that woman's smaller brain, her physical weakness, and her gentle nature unfitted her for medical study" (Bonner 1992: 11).

32. For one exposition of the argument that man is the hunter and woman the childbearer and -rearer, see Tiger (1970: 60), who asserts:

"There are differences in methods of locomotion between males and females, in the ability to throw spears, bolas, rocks, etc., in adaptability to temperature changes presumably related to hunting; males show greater spatial-geographical ability, they are more aggressive, etc.—these are all differences which relate more clearly (or as clearly) to differences in activities like hunting and defense than to childbearing and rearing . . . I take the existence of these differences to be an indication and outcome of the process of human evolution." And again (67): "Given the overwhelming portion of human history in which females' chief functions have been maternal, it was presumably advantageous for females to be closely and uninhibitedly attuned to their young. For males this responsiveness could be a disadvantage beyond the point at which it does not interfere with political and economic activities."

33. E.g., Gilligan (1982); Chodorow (1978); Noddings (1984); Belenky, Field, Clinchy, Goldberger, and Tarule (1986).

34. Kessler and McKenna (1978) advance a powerful critique of such binary comparisons, noting that we cannot talk about differences without classifying the incumbents of the two categories under comparison. Thus, in order to compare "women" and "men," we must already know what women and men are, and who belongs to each category. Among biologists, social scientists, and behavioral scientists, *classification precedes comparison*, the basis for classification being the "incorrigible proposition" that humans are "naturally" divided into two genders.

35. West and Zimmerman (1987); Coltrane (1989); Ginsburg and Tsing (1990); DeVault (1991); Unger (1989).

36. Marjorie DeVault notes: "Doing gender . . . is not just an individual performance, but an interactional process, a process of collective production and recognition of 'adequate' women and men through concerted activity" (1991: 118).

37. Ginsburg and Tsing explain: "By 'gender' we mean the ways a society organizes people into male and female categories and the ways meanings are produced around these categories . . . Gender is not seen as fixed or 'natural' but rather as a category subject to change and specifically to *negotiation*. As ethnographers, we pay attention to the ways in which people learn, accept, negotiate, and resist the categories of 'difference' that define and constrain them in everyday life" (1991: 2).

38. Such gut reactions related to gender are evident in accounts of cadets' ferocious harassment of the first group of women at the Citadel, and the slow reaction of college officials to incidents involving setting women cadets on fire, circulating obscene photographs, and so forth (e.g., *New York Times*, January 22, 1997: A8).

39. Bourdieu (1977, 1984, 1990a, 1990b).

40. "Socialization tends to constitute the body as an analogical operator establishing all sorts of practical equivalences between the different divisions of the social world—divisions between the sexes, between the age groups, and between the social classes—or, more precisely, between the meanings and values associated with the individuals occupying practically equivalent positions in the spaces defined by these divisions . . . It does so by integrating the symbolism of social domination and submission and the symbolism of sexual domination and submission into the same body language" (Bourdieu 1984: 475).

41. Thus, I noticed that seven of the thirty-three women surgeons I studied had poor posture, as did two more women surgical residents whom I did not spend much time with. I know this means *something*, but I am unable to say exactly what. Their bearing struck me because it was so different from that of the male surgeons I studied. Here's a description of one from my fieldnotes:

    "She looked fresh, attractive, not wildly beautiful, but kind of cute. Except for one thing: during the day, I noticed that she has abysmal posture; there are all these men surgeons standing straight, like that Shakespeare character, astride the world; and these women with terrible posture; how many can I remember [I list several]. Not all, but still . . . The only male surgeon I can think of offhand with poor posture was that house officer who worked for [a chief of general surgery in the 1980s], who he wasn't sure would make a surgeon, and indeed did leave surgery. It says something about self-image, for the men and the women."

    These women's bodies tell me something about self-image and about self-confidence. But exactly what do they tell me? My body knows, but I can't seem to translate that knowledge into words.

42. "There is a contingent, though not arbitrary, relation between the male body and masculinity and the female body and femininity. To claim this is neither biologism nor essentialism but is rather to acknowledge the importance of complex and ubiquitous networks of

signification to the historically, psychologically, and culturally variable ways of being a man or a woman" (Gatens 1996: 13).

43. Judith Lorber's discussion of "dismantling Noah's Ark" exemplifies such a program of planned change (Lorber 1994: 291–304). Because she approaches gender as a *social institution*, disregarding its embodied aspects, I am convinced that her program (in the unlikely event that it were implemented) would not eradicate difference, nor would it abolish what she describes as men's emotional and sexual exploitation based on that difference. Lorber contrasts a belief in "natural" or biological differences with the social construction of differentiated gender categories: the (untrue) belief is used to mystify the gender categories; the gender categories are used to exploit women. This either/or contrast ignores *embodied* difference, which may indeed be changed—but not overnight. Feminist philosopher Moira Gatens is committed, as is Lorber, to altering the power imbalance between men and women. But her subtle and nuanced analysis accepts the fact that because differences are embodied, change must be gradual: "To say that our 'natures' are constructed is not to say that we have the freedom to become anything we like . . . This illusion arises from paying insufficient attention to the embodiedness of this nature. Our embodied history cannot be thrown off as if it were a coat that one has donned only involuntarily in the first place. Whether we like it or not, in so far as our values and our 'ways of being' are embodied they cannot be wished away or dismissed by a pure act of will" (Gatens 1996: 105).

44. Comparing West and Fenstermaker's analyses of race, class, and gender to Bourdieu's powerful yet subtle approach to social difference points up the inadequacies of this disembodied social constructionist approach (Bourdieu 1984; see also West and Zimmerman 1987).

45. The concept of "habitus" illuminates and enriches social constructionist analyses based on "doing" or "negotiating" gender. The constructionist analyses have explanatory power; I would have difficulty understanding and explaining my findings without them. But they can generate problems. When gender is presented as an interactional process, a category subject to negotiation and change, we may be easily beguiled by what Bourdieu calls the "occasionalist illusion" (1977: 81): we may assume that gender inheres solely in the interaction or situation and that, consequently, altering the interaction or

situation will alter gender. Rejecting explanations based on innate "deep structure" does not necessarily make such phenomena shallow. When we think about the opposition between "masculinity" and "femininity" as a "fundamental principle of division of the social and symbolic world" (Bourdieu 1990a: 78), then the doing of gender is seen to be far deeper and more powerful than an explanation based solely upon interaction might suggest. In this view, gender is an aspect of an embodied "logic of practice" prior to thought, resistant to reason. We learn gender before we learn speech; we do gender before we think abstractly.

The concept of "habitus" is more parsimonious and powerful than social constructionist theories. Thus, although social constructionist approaches may focus on the body—often with great insight—*embodiment* is not an integral part of the theory (e.g., Fine and Macpherson 1992; Brodkey and Fine 1992; E. Martin 1991: 131). Instead, bodies are often presented as battlefields, on and through which social politics are negotiated (e.g., Fine 1992: 27–29; Rapp 1990).

In addition, discussions of "doing" or "negotiating" gender tend to ignore the passage of time or treat it too lightly. When gender is conceptualized as an "interactional achievement," analyses tend to concentrate on the here and now (e.g., West and Zimmerman 1987; Coltrane 1989; DeVault 1991). Time is not an intrinsic part of social constructionist explanations. Unlike the habitus, which is a dialectic process based on *interaction through time,* social constructionist analyses must first bring in the passage of time before addressing it. Moira Gatens recognizes the significance of the passage of time, and notes the importance of attending to "the history of social bodies and their practices and the manner in which these practices actually institute and perpetuate differential forms of embodiment (1996: 98–99); she advocates "a historical, or genealogical, approach to understanding the specificity of social, political and ethical relations *as they are embodied* in this or that community or culture (1996: 105).

Difference is not an integral part of social constructionist theory either; "categories of difference," yes, but the emphasis is on the social categories rather than on difference per se. Feminist difference theorists have been criticized for paying too little attention to differences among women. Ginsburg and Tsing (1990: 3–5) discuss what they call "the challenge of diversity" to feminist and anthropological theory; their postmodernist solution is to attend to "competing discourses, divergent forms of consciousness, and modes of resistance to oppressive circumstances," to show how gender is variously produced in a variety of social sites. The authors examine "categories of difference," recognizing that these are multiple and cross-cutting, and can be mobilized in strategic fashion by individuals and groups.

Yet despite the fact that such theorizing may be sensitive to differences among women, *difference is not intrinsic to the theory.* This may pose problems. By insisting on diversity as a political as well as methodological requirement, such analyses can lead to infinite splitting. Women differ from men. African-American women differ from white women. White working-class women differ from white middle- and upper-class women. Older women differ from younger women, lesbians from heterosexuals, and so forth. An overenthusiastic rejection of "false generalization," may thus lead to a certain unwillingness to generalize at all, except within certain predetermined and politically acceptable categories, thus stifling social research (J. R. Martin 1994: 646–647; see also Bordo 1993: 238–239).

Another problem is the assumption of flexibility involved when one investigates how social processes produce, challenge, or confirm gender categories (Ginsburg and Tsing 1990: 5). Yes, flexibility exists, and gender can be negotiated—but always within certain well-defined constraints. The categories, discourses, symbolism, forms of consciousness, activities, and meanings of gender differ among different social groups and classes, and no amount of "negotiation" will transform the embodied categories associated with one social classification into those of another.

Difference is central to the concept of "habitus," which encompasses and explains differences between members of different social groups and classes, as well as gender differences between members of the same group; consequently, it allows us to avoid assuming that all women are the same. We can also avoid the fears of false generalization, which encourage a fragmenting rhetoric of diversity and render all social generalizations suspect.

## 3. Telling Stories

1. Tedlock argues that the classic anthropological research method, *participant observation*, has shifted in the past twenty years to a more inclusive and interesting technique, *the observation of participation*.

Rather than merely observing the people being studied, the anthropologist apprehends and observes her (or his) own and others' *co-participation* within the ethnographic encounter. All pretense at being transparent or invisible evaporates. Instead, the researcher's role expands from that of observer to actor: she observes herself interacting with the host people. This shift in research method generates a "transformation" in representation. The anthropologist is no longer forced to choose between writing a memoir focused on the *self* (herself and her experiences) or a standard monograph focused on the *other* (those studied). Instead, she can present the dialogue between self and other in a single "narrative ethnography."

2. E.g., Briggs (1970); Myerhoff (1974, 1979); Favret-Saada (1980); Kondo (1990); Narayan (1989); Lavie (1990); Brown (1991); Behar (1993); Abu-Lughod (1993). In addition, vivid accounts have been published by nonanthropologist wives who accompanied their husbands into the field; for an examination of the marital division of textual labor, see Tedlock (1995).

3. James Clifford (1986: 15) describes men's dialogical accounts as "an inscription of communicative processes that exist, historically, between subjects in relations of power." Deborah Gordon (1988) is the first of many who have criticized Clifford's explanations (in his Introduction, where his laudatory quote about experimental dialogical anthropology appears) of why no feminists were invited to the seminar that formed the basis of the book *Writing Culture: The Poetics and Politics of Ethnography* (1986). Gordon (1988: 7–8) was also the first to note the now-notorious photographic cover of the volume: in the foreground is conference participant Stephen Tyler in the field (India), bent over a pad, writing; behind him is the smaller figure of a dark-skinned man observing the white male anthropologist; barely visible in the background is a diminutive blurred figure, a dark-skinned woman holding a child. "The graphic design of the cover includes a thick black line running through her eyes, which cuts off her gaze."

The cover of *Writing Culture*, then, is inadvertently diagnostic of the poetics and politics of an anthropological canon that emphasizes the work of white men, while diminishing the stature of minority men and obscuring and graphically concealing the subjectivity of women.

4. The methodological views and practices of Barbara Tedlock and her

husband, Dennis, are sufficiently controversial to have incited a ferocious attack, at the December 1994 meetings of the American Anthropological Association, by a group of prominent senior anthropologists, who attempted to oust the Tedlocks from their joint editorship of the association's flagship journal, *American Anthropologist*.

5. Paul Stoller, who writes narrative ethnographies about his fieldwork in Africa (Stoller and Olkes 1987; Stoller 1989a, 1989b), quotes publishers' comments on his work (1989a: 28–29): "Both reviewers thought that the script contained some interesting data, but felt that the theoretical argument was insufficiently well developed"; "What kind of contribution does this piece make to ethnological theory, method, compared to other works on the topic?"; "The weakness of its theoretical grounding leads to the lack of any real integration of the descriptive material."

I have received similar comments from manuscript and book reviewers: "Long on description, short on analysis"; "I did not like the omnipresence of the writer in the book . . . This book is probably not suitable for a university press. It might find a commercial audience as the diary of an insider but would not likely be used in university classes"; "I would have appreciated more interpretive and theoretical work."

6. Of the ten women surgeons I've heard outline these alternatives, Dr. Krieger's explanations were the simplest, clearest, and easiest for a terrified woman to remember.

7. The interview was tape-recorded. I've condensed it slightly to remove extraneous details. For those who have difficulty understanding surgeon-speak, I provide a "translation" below. My thanks to Fanny Kasher, M.D., who helped render the technical concepts and terms into easily understandable English.

> *Dr. Krieger:* Toward the end of my chief residency I stopped coping . . . After so many years I just started to understand that no matter what I did, it wasn't going to work. I was never going to be equal, and I was never going to be looked at equally. There was one particular incident that sort of set this thing off . . . I think one of the reasons I had such a hard time is because I really thought, *I truly believed* for a number of years, that if I just worked hard and did right that I would be equal. That there was no way I would be denied. That I would just—I would just

prove that I was as good as anybody else and they would *have* to believe that. And that was proved to be a lie.

*Anthropologist:* What was the incident?

*Dr. Krieger:* [It] happened in the spring of my chief residency . . . I was chief resident at the Veteran's Administration Hospital, and the chief residents in the VA took calls from home [when something happened, they called the residents to come in]. And I was covering one weekend, and the second-year resident called me at home . . . in the middle of the afternoon on Saturday to say, panicked—this was a not very talented second-year resident—panicked, because he said to me, "There's a guy in the emergency room and his belly is wide open, with his guts hanging out." I said, "Okay, who operated on him?" I figured he'd broken all the layers of stitches from a recent operation. He said, "He wasn't operated on, but he's wide open." I said, "Okay, Chuck, calm down, I'll be right there." Because clearly I'm not going to get any information from this guy over the phone . . . I put my shoes on and I walked over. And sure enough, there was this poor old vet in the emergency room with his guts hanging out of a hole in his belly. And what basically had happened is, this was a guy with very, very bad alcoholic damage to his liver who had very bad fluid collection in the belly from the alcoholic damage. And he had had an umbilical hernia, a weakened area of the abdominal wall from the fluid buildup—this is something that is recognized happens occasionally: hernias break open occasionally when there is fluid buildup. This weakened area broke open at home, and some of his guts came out and they sort of sat there for a couple of days drying out. And he came out of his alcoholic stupor long enough to show up at the VA. It also turns out that he had an extensive medical history—had had open-heart surgery, his chest had been opened for surgery— and now his guts are hanging out. So we got the guy admitted to the hospital—clearly he was going to need to go to the operating room—got him moved up to the Intensive Care Unit, and we're getting ready to prepare to take him to the operating room. I asked the second-year resident to do some appropriate things, including putting in a heart catheter for monitoring, and a urine catheter, and all kinds of other jazz. And I went off to start to marshal the forces to come in. At the VA, this is a big deal. Nobody's there. We had to open the operating room on a Saturday. In the VA, you needed an act of Congress to do this! So I called up the nursing staff and I called anesthesia and I called the attending [the senior surgeon who was supervising on call], and I said, "There's a guy, I think he's popped an umbilical hernia," and I gave him the whole story. So the attending said to me, "Okay, fix it." I said, "Do you have any other advice?" [laughter] "No, no, just fix it." I said, "Well, I figured that out already, thank you very much." And I hung up the phone. The second-year resident was having a tough time putting the catheter into the heart chamber because the guy had scarring along the entry areas from his previous surgery, and also he was *very* dehydrated at this point, which collapsed his veins and made them hard to locate. [Intestines lying outside the body for two days become dried out, dead, and infected. This is a true emergency, where the patient is in imminent danger of dying.] So I went there . . . and I got the catheter in. While we're waiting for the OR to be opened, we get a chest X-ray. He has a small a small collection of air in the lung from the catheter insertion. Okay, that's okay, it happens. [It's a minor complication that can occur in such situations. A chest tube corrects the problem.] We put a chest tube in. He's perfectly fine. We go to the operating room. The second-year resident falls asleep; I have to throw him out of the OR. I open the abdomen. He has liters and liters and liters of fluid and terrible liver damage. I drain the fluid, I remove the dead area of bowel, I put it back together. I trim off the damaged areas of abdominal wall, which is all black from all 'his stuff hangin' out, tie the deep layers of abdominal wall back together real tight so the same thing won't happen again, and take him to the ICU. And lo and behold, ten days later the guy's well enough to be off my service: he's on the rehab service, perfectly healed!

*Anthropologist:* It's a miracle.

*Dr. Krieger:* A miracle. And it's an interesting case. And it went well. I presented the case at an M & M conference that we had [a weekly Mortality and Morbidity conference where cases resulting in complications or deaths are presented and discussed], and I thought, "This is a great case."

*Anthropologist:* It's really pretty cool, yes.

*Dr. Krieger:* This is pretty impressive—this is a great case! But the chairman was not there that day, and the rounds were being run by the next most senior attending . . . I presented this history. So the first thing they did, they spent fifteen minutes torturing me over this insignificant air in the lung: "What had happened?" "What was the lighting?" "What was the this?" "What was the that?" The guy was dehydrated—had no veins to put the catheter into—and he was scarred from his heart surgery, and he had every possible reason to get this relatively common complication. And I took full responsibility—never mentioned the other resident involved. But, you know, I just didn't get it—I didn't get why this was such a big deal. Then we moved on. Then they wanted to talk about the performance of the surgery, and one of the senior attendings raised his hand and said, Why didn't I bring the ends of the intestines out of the body to form a stoma? Why did I put it back together again? Why didn't I bring the ends out? I said, well, the patient had massive fluid—that's a relative contraindication to bringing out the ends of the intestines to form a stoma. Plus the fact this was proximal small bowel; there was no reason not to reconnect the ends internally in this setting. It wasn't pus in the abdomen—it was just fluid. And I basically justified myself medically. And his response was, "Well, *if* it had been just a little small bowel, *if* there was massive fluid, you should have brought the ends out." I'm like, "Yeah, well, so big deal." So that was another ten minutes. Now the last thing is, the senior attending who's running rounds says to me—I'm still standing up there, I've been there twenty minutes now, and this is not going well, I'm sensing that this is not going well—he says to me, "Well, after you closed the abdomen, did you leave the skin open?" And I said, "Well, we cleaned up the abdominal wall. We closed the deep layers of the abdomen and left the skin open." He said, "Did he leak fluid through his closure?" I said, "No." He said, "Wait a minute—he didn't leak at all?" I said, "No, he didn't," which was the absolute truth. He said, "Well, the last patient that I closed with massive fluid leaked terribly through the wound." I said, "Well this patient didn't leak." So he concluded the discussion by saying, "Well, I guess I'd rather be lucky than smart."

*Anthropologist:* That son-of-a-bitch!

*Dr. Krieger:* And then I knew. And then I had that flash. And I said—the way I commented on this afterwards when I reported this incident to everybody who would stand still long enough to hear the story—I said, you know, "If I reported at M & M that I had resurrected Lazarus, they would ask me why I'd waited four days!"

8. According to a surgeon-informant, this particular life-threatening complication, post-operative bleeding, "would be viewed by some of us as [indicating] hasty or shoddy surgery."

9. In some ways, the field of breast surgery resembles that of matrimonial law, which also has a pool of female practitioners. Both can be emotionally charged. Breast surgeons and divorce lawyers are haunted by telephone calls from distraught female patients and clients; the substantive content of the calls is usually less significant than the terror and sorrow motivating them. Patients and clients demand emotional support. They devour time. Many surgeons and lawyers prefer to avoid such emotional demands, especially since (or perhaps because) breast surgery and matrimonial law are both low in the professional prestige ranking when compared, for example, to the martial specialties of head-and-neck surgery or trial litigation.

10. A fourth surgeon had an unusually compassionate nurse who spent a lot of time talking to patients. The nurse herself had undergone breast surgery; she told me that, when she was forty-one, a male surgeon had said to her, "At your age, what do you need your breast for?"—an experience similar to ones recounted to me by other women. She and I agreed that no male surgeon would ever say to a man, even one in his nineties, "At your age, what do you need your testicle for?"

11. During the third and fourth years of medical school, students leave the classroom for hospital "clerkships" or "clinical rotations" in various specialties. During this time, they learn basic skills and are ex-

posed to diverse career options. Like Dr. Krieger, they often discover that they dislike a projected career choice and enjoy a specialty they thought they would hate.

## 4. Women Leading

1. The anesthesiologist and I were at the head of the table. As usual, I stood on a stool, so that I could observe what was happening without getting in anyone's way.
2. This undoubtedly applies to a variety of situations and occupations. Surgery, however, is the profession I have observed and am most familiar with. Moreover, such phenomena are more dramatic and visible in an embodied occupation with relatively few women practitioners.
3. Patients, colleagues, and superiors also react differently. These reactions will be examined in subsequent chapters.
4. Women in surgical leadership positions exist but are relatively rare. I studied three: the celebrated surgeon in the first vignette, a full professor in a university department of surgery; another woman who had been chief of surgery at a university hospital; and a third, who before going into semiretirement had been head of a subspecialty department of surgery.
5. This excerpt and all the following unattributed quotations come from tape-recorded interviews with the women I studied.
6. This woman had a superb ability to do gender without compromising her intelligence, ability, and drive. Small and curvy, with enormous eyes and a warm bubbly manner, she had been head of the cheerleader squad in high school, and had belonged to a sorority in college, while earning a degree in chemical engineering—the only woman in the chemical engineering program.
7. This appeared in a section of the newsletter called "Resident's Corner." It was surrounded by quotation marks, so I am assuming it was a letter. A year earlier, after a description of my research was published in the *Newsletter of the Association of Women Surgeons*, I received a phone call from a distraught female surgery resident in California, who described the same problem and asked for advice. Subsequently, after discussing these issues as a member of a panel on

leadership at a meeting of the Association of Women Surgeons, I was thanked by a young woman: "I thought I was the only one!" said this attractive young intern.

8. I was amused that the newsletter's response to this query defined this resident's difficulties as a "communication gap." The advice, however, was very similar to the behavior elicited by the nurses, which I am about to describe.

9. The sexual component of this problem will be discussed in Chapter 5.

10. I have observed a few male nurses interact with surgeons. One suggested that I study male nurses. This man interacted with other people on a more equal footing than the female nurses did: he joined a female chief resident and myself in the cafeteria with no invitation and subsequently dominated the conversation; he assumed a "joking relationship" with residents, teasing the men and initiating a kind of deferential flirting with the women. In addition, unlike female nurses, he asked questions about surgical maneuvers in the OR. This man thought the status of male nurses was analogous to that of female surgeons. The status is *comparable,* but not *analogous:* the career patterns of male and female nurses, their status, and their relationships with peers and superiors differ. Male nurses and male surgeons have an advantage (see Floge and Merrill 1985).

11. Three of the women had been nurses before attending medical school and then being trained as a surgeon; another had been a physiotherapist. Several had mothers who were former nurses. A surgeon's daughter described how her mother, who had been a nurse, encouraged her to obtain medical rather than nursing training.

12. I do not wish to portray nurses as husband-hunting airheads or hostile bitches. Many are extraordinarily competent, intelligent, and sympathetic to women surgeons. But nurses frequently behave differently toward men and women in authority—especially *young* women in authority. Discussing the supportive/subversive attitude of nurses, one woman surgeon said, "They want you to succeed, and yet. . . .," while another noted that she had to tread a narrow line with nurses: she couldn't be too soft or they'd walk all over her; she couldn't be too domineering or they'd resent and resist. "It's a tightrope," she concluded. Men are not required to perform this balancing act.

13. I am indebted to Roy Mendelsohn, M.D., for the phrase and the concept "the dark side of envy."

14. Thus, the secretary to the chief of surgery made her vicious remark only after a powerful protector had withdrawn his support, exposing the resident to attack. As for the senior woman, she quit her prestigious position after a highly politicized battle with a dishonest surgeon with powerful protectors whom she had attempted to curb. It would not surprise me to learn that the director of nursing was aware of this factional conflict when she challenged the senior woman.

## 5. Forging the Iron Surgeon

1. In fact, the man exists: every surgeon to whom I've mentioned the details has instantly identified the chief and his program.

2. Scrub suits have additional advantages. Worn with sneakers or clogs, they are far more comfortable than street clothing—especially women's street clothing—for the ten- to sixteen-hour surgical day. Residents' clothing often gets soiled from messy procedures, and scrubs go into a bin at the end of the day (the hospital is responsible for laundering them). Moreover, wearing scrubs around the hospital immediately identifies one as a member of the OR team.

3. Let me emphasize that all this is hearsay. I made no effort to substantiate or discredit these rumors; whether they were true or not, they indicated a climate of fear. Let me also emphasize that the people who related these stories all indicated that this man had transformed a lackluster department and training program into one of the most highly respected surgical programs in the country. I was never introduced to the chief and never learned whether he was aware of my presence in the hospitals he supervised. I kept a very low profile, fearing he might prohibit his surgeons from cooperating with my research. I must admit that I rather enjoyed perceiving him as a shadowy, somewhat threatening, paradigmatic surgical presence: the iron surgeon who forged others in his image.

4. Reviewing a book on the Libby Zion case—in which an eighteen-year-old drug-addicted patient died after being treated by a (possibly) sleep-deprived intern in internal medicine, and the patient's journalist father mounted a relentless legal and media-based campaign against the hospital—Rothman (1996: 32) notes that as a result

of the publicity surrounding the case, residency training throughout the country was transformed, with accrediting groups insisting on less crushing schedules for trainees. He indicates, however, that surgical training has successfully resisted all pressures for change, despite the fact that the "crushing" schedules that were ameliorated involved residents' being on call every third or fourth night, whereas surgeons—whose schedules were unaltered—are required to be on call every second or third night.

5. Some general-surgery programs take five years; others take longer, including a required year (or more) of research. After finishing a training program, a surgeon may obtain a fellowship for advanced training. A cardiothoracic surgeon I studied spent eleven years being trained—a period that included various prestigious fellowships.

6. This excerpt from my fieldnotes was followed by a passage in which I wondered how recent developments in the field of medicine (see Chapter 9) might affect this mystique: "Does this attitude toward time change when doctors and patients become interchangeable mass-production cogs? Yes, time is then divided into prescheduled units—just as disease care is divided into units, and patients and doctors are divided into units. We have rationalization and bureaucratization of medicine. The price: carpal tunnel (or thoracic outlet) syndrome of the soul. Human beings aren't meant to function that way. Both systems deform (or preform); but the first carries the concept of the hero, where people do more than they rationally can (although the hero pays a price for this).

7. In this public hospital, which served impoverished patients who could not afford private medical care, residents were accorded a great deal of autonomy in deciding upon and performing procedures. Although senior ENT and general surgeons came in to help and supervise, the procedures were performed primarily by residents.

8. See Kanter (1977a: 206–242; 1977b). As more women are accepted into surgical programs, this may change. But the proportion of women in a surgical program is just one of the elements that affect the objective and subjective experiences of trainees; individual and institutionalized sexism are also important. To give just one example, a program that does not offer separate dressing rooms and on-call rooms for women will make female trainees feel like uncomfortable

exceptions, no matter how many women are exposed to these conditions.

Moreover, the increase in the number of women in surgical training programs has been slow, and is disproportionately concentrated in certain programs rather than being spread across the board. Of the thirty-two women surgeons with whom I conducted tape-recorded interviews, seven said there were no other women in their training programs. Others, when asked about women in their program, gave responses such as the following:

"I was the first woman to complete my surgical residency program. There was a woman a year ahead of me who got fired at the end of my first year there. There were other women who came in years after I did, but there were none ahead of me."

"No, I was the only one, until my fourth year."

"I think there were two women in the program ahead of me. And the program director, after I had been there a couple of years, told me that if I hadn't worked out, they were never going to have any other women, because they disliked the women they had had in the program so much, before me.

9. The following descriptions of what it was like to be a female resident come from tape-recorded interviews.

10. In contrast to the catch-as-catch-can American system, maternity leave is guaranteed by law in Canada. Every pregnant employee receives two-thirds of her salary for six months. If she wishes to stay home with the child, her employers must hold her position for five years. In addition, fathers are permitted to take six months of unpaid maternity leave.

11. Rogers, Kunkel, and Field (1994) interviewed a cohort of psychiatric residents about their attitudes toward pregnant peers. Although psychiatric programs are not as demanding as surgical ones, they encountered similar resentment among some residents.

12. For many procedures, the Occupational Safety and Health Administration now requires surgeons to wear waterproof gowns and spectacles, to keep from being splashed with blood from patients who might have AIDS. The senior woman told me she hated the specs, but she wore them. At the time, I wondered whether the refusal to wear specs was macho behavior on Dr. Callahan's part.

13. I am indebted to Sue-Ellen Jacobs for this phrase and concept.

14. I did not pay attention to ethno-religious background when I began this study. Only when I noticed the number of women who had been brought up in Catholic families did I go back to the surgeons I had already studied and ask them about their family's religious background. The numbers surprised me *and* the surgeons I studied.

15. When I learned of the existence of an Orthodox Jewish woman surgeon, I recruited her for the study precisely because of her religious background.

16. It would be helpful to compare these proportions with the proportions of male surgeons raised as Catholics and as Jews, and with the proportions of Catholic and Jewish male and female internists and medical students. No comparable figures are available. A demographer who works for the American Medical Association told me that government regulations prohibit such inquiries.

17. If this analysis is correct, the present scarcity of nuns in the United States may influence achievement patterns among Catholic women.

18. I admit that, since my sample was so small, the following discussion is highly speculative. It's conceivable that I'm projecting upon the surgeons my own personal reactions to the choices they must make, and that my feeling of utter visceral certainty about this analysis says more about me than about the women surgeons.

19. I am speaking now of *culture,* not religion. Other groups (e.g., Italians, Greeks, Jamaicans) possess a similar relation to food; many, however, do not.

20. Among Orthodox Jews, the child of a Jewish mother and *any* father is automatically Jewish, whereas the child of a Jewish father and non-Jewish mother must undergo conversion to become Jewish.

21. An article celebrating the value and regretting the loss of female domestic rituals appeared recently in *Commentary* (Lichter 1994). Although it was published in a Jewish magazine, its author attempts to trace the value of these rituals to the Victorian home—an interesting example of blindness on her part and on the part of the secular Jewish editors of the journal. Like so many aspects of culture, the Jewish female ethos is taken for granted to such an extent that it is almost invisible to secular Jews.

22. Despite the fact that she downplayed these qualities, the Dr. Carlsen possessed strength, stamina, intelligence, and a driving will. Without these attributes, she could never have completed the surgical train-

ing program, much less have had a miscarriage and a baby during the same period.

## 6. The Gender of Care

1. Because this patient was pregnant, she did not receive intravenous sedation and no anesthesiologist was present. Most of the other biopsies I observed this surgeon perform were on sedated patients, who slept through most of the procedure.
2. Linguist Deborah Tannen (1990: 67) indicates that women are more likely to share information, whereas men frequently use information as a weapon in a struggle for status: "If women are focusing on connections, they will be motivated to minimize the difference in expertise and be as comprehensible as possible. Since their goal is to maintain the appearance of similarity and equal status, sharing knowledge helps to even the score. Their tone of voice sends metamessages of support rather than disdain . . . If a man focuses on the negotiation of status and feels someone must have the upper hand, he may feel more comfortable when he has it. His attunement to the fact that having more information, knowledge, or skill puts him in a one-up position comes through in his way of talking."
3. I do not think this was necessarily conscious or intentional behavior; putting themselves on the patient's level was an almost instinctive way of relating for some women. Having dinner with this surgeon after completing my observations, I told her that I admired the way she shared her knowledge and tried to avoid hierarchy, even to kneeling down to the patient's level to make eye contact. She responded, "If you asked me whether I did that, I'd deny it!"
4. During rounds, this woman said to the other residents: "The trouble with rounding [making rounds] in the afternoon is that they're all awake!" I noted in my fieldnotes: "She is a surgeon, an orthopedic surgeon . . . I once heard [another orthopedist] talk like that. It's not a question of niceness, but of how they define their mission. Her mission is caring for the patient's bones and any other part of their anatomy that falls within the purview of an orthopedist."
5. Perri Klass, in her book on attending medical school (Klass 1987), describes the process of absorbing the culture of medicine as "a not entirely benign procedure." Such training begins during the clinical

years, the last two years of medical school, and continues through the residency. The process is not entirely benign in any medical specialty, but is especially long, difficult, and concentrated (one might even say "malignant") in surgery.

6. This is not strictly correct. The surgeon did talk to one patient, who had some cookies on the table near her bed: she asked about them, said wistfully that she had a sweet tooth, was offered a cookie, took it, and discussed the recipe with the patient.

7. This surgeon asked if the patient wanted her to "remove the cyst liquid," rather than inquiring whether the patient wanted her to "aspirate" the cyst. Unlike the less compassionate surgeons, she routinely used phrases that patients could understand.

8. This would involve a basic alteration in the iron-surgeon ethos. Whether such a change is likely, I do not know. Surgery—indeed, medicine in general—is changing so rapidly that the future is murky. One possibility is an increase in bureaucratization and commodification of patient care, with interchangeable doctors being assigned fixed slots of time to care for interchangeable patients. In such a future, both compassion and technical competence will diminish.

## 7. A Greedy Institution

1. A senior surgeon who presented annual "commendations" to residents had in three succeeding years bestowed on this man the "Hands of Wood," "Hands of Cement," and "Captain Blood" awards. (Another hapless resident who had almost killed a patient with an overdose of insulin was given the "Claus von Bülow Award.")

2. In fact, the man who hired her at the Health Maintenance Organization was another exemplary surgeon, whose technique, clinical judgment, and moral probity were universally admired. He hated thinking about money, and preferred a situation where he could do what he wished for patients without having to worry about financial details.

3. In the medical prestige system, academic physicians rank highest (although this may be denied by private practitioners); then come those in private or group practice; below these are salaried physi-

cians, hired by an individual physician, group, hospital, or HMO; and at the lowest rung are part-time salaried physicians.

4. All of these women were married to physicians. In one case, the employer used this as an argument, when he told the woman that he had to provide for his wife and his retirement, while she could rely on her husband.

5. This quotation and the following one come from tape-recorded interviews.

6. *Divided Lives* (Walsh 1995: 189–259) describes the experiences of Dr. Alison Estabrook, an academic surgeon at Columbia-Presbyterian Medical Center, who discovered that her starting salary was $40,000 a year less than men who had been hired from her residency class. Trained as a general surgeon, Estabrook was steered into breast surgery by the head of general surgery. She was then promised the position of chief of the breast service, a promise that was broken, as the department attempted to recruit several senior men. After a long, exhausting struggle, just when Estabrook was ready to move to another institution, she was offered the job of permanent chief of the breast service.

7. Similar phenomena have been reported for women in every branch of academia (Aisenberg and Harrington 1988).

8. An article in *Archives of Surgery* (Kemeny 1993) describes the career of Nina Starr Braunwald, a pioneer who helped create the specialty of cardiac surgery. Married to a medical-school classmate, Braunwald moved several times during her residency and surgical career, following her husband, who was offered increasingly prestigious jobs. Despite a grueling full-time schedule, during which time she developed and implanted the first successful prosthetic heart valve, she had three children. After a number of moves, Braunwald followed her husband to Harvard Medical School, where he was offered a position as department chair. Harvard offered Braunwald an assistant professorship, which she was able to negotiate upward to associate professor. She spent the final twenty years of her career as an associate professor, despite having published 115 articles and numerous book chapters, and despite having made vital contributions to the field of cardiac surgery.

9. Let me emphasize that I mean exactly what I say: *I never saw this*. My experience, however, is limited: I studied few senior women.

Whether there is little Queen Bee behavior in surgery today, as compared to fields in which there are more women, or whether I did not study enough women in senior positions to come across this phenomenon, I cannot tell.

10. An issue I scrupulously did *not* investigate was the sexual orientation of the unmarried women. Although during my research I was introduced to one resident who publicly identified herself as a lesbian, as does the celebrated breast surgeon Dr. Susan Love, none of the women I studied so identified themselves. I felt that sexual orientation had little to do with the kind of surgeon a woman was, and that moreover it was information that might cause difficulties for someone in a conservative profession such as surgery.

11. When studying general surgeons, I learned that many were married to former nurses (Cassell 1991). During my later study of women surgeons, I found that many male surgical residents had also married nurses. Unfortunately, I have no statistics on this.

12. During the course of my research, I met two academic women surgeons who each had four children and who are now chairs of specialty departments. Observing these women in action will teach women trainees far more about how to be an effective but not necessarily iron surgeon, and far more about how best to conduct their professional and personal lives, than could ever be garnered from books, lectures, or feminist admonitions.

13. In point of fact, Dr. Travis married soon after this session was held.

14. The Association of Women Surgeons (414 Plaza Drive, Suite 209, Westmont, Illinois 60559) has a mentoring program and a first-rate booklet, *The Pocket Mentor*, with advice for women residents. I think there should be institutional mechanisms as well, set up by medical schools and departments of surgery.

15. My relatively optimistic view is not the only possible scenario. A noted woman surgeon, who read this book in manuscript, commented:

"Perhaps she should be asked to think about the alternative possibility: . . . that with managed care, there will be far fewer women entering surgical disciplines.

"I believe (and I can be as wrong as she may well be proved right) that the structure of medicine in the United States is rapidly moving to a two-tiered configuration. In a rush to provide primary-care doctors (a scarce commodity, we are told) women have been admitted to medical schools in numbers almost equal to those of men. The bulk of these women will end up in a primary-care discipline and for a precious few years will be in a position to dictate the terms of their employment. However, eventually they will form the bottom tier, of ultimately low prestige and pay, in medicine. In answer to studies that find too many specialists in the U.S. (both in medicine and surgery), training programs for these specialists are being drastically cut. A surgical department chair (such chairs are virtually all men at the present time) who once had four resident slots to fill per year now finds his program has been cut to two. Before, he could 'waste' a slot on a woman (who, horrors, might get married or pregnant). With the smaller allotted numbers, his choices for residents will most likely be clones of himself. My guess is that we will see a drastic reduction in the number of women entering surgery over the next ten years, and that the second, more prestigious tier of medicine will be composed mostly of male surgeons and medical specialists who will enjoy enhanced professional stature and high incomes because they will have become the scarce commodity. Without appreciable numbers of women to taint their world, they will be the ones to retain and maintain power and control of the medical world, especially in the academic medical centers where most tertiary care will be clustered."

## 8. A Worst-case Scenario

1. Mead (1968: 208); Murphy and Murphy (1974: 107–108); Gregor (1985: 100–104).
2. She was the fourth woman to graduate from the surgical training program, including the subspecialty divisions.
3. This comes from a tape-recorded interview, in response to a question asking her to tell how it happened that she had become a doctor. Unless identified as from my fieldnotes, all extended quotations come from this interview.
4. In the "match" system, medical students interview in the specialty of their choice, then rank the programs they are most interested in. At the same time, the training programs rank the students. Students'

rankings and program rankings are then compared and weighted to yield the final decision as to who goes where.

5. She was the one who got up to care for the baby on the alternate nights when she was home, she said, because her anesthesiologist husband, who suffered from insomnia, had difficulty falling asleep once he was awakened. To help with childcare, her mother-in-law moved to the same city. Dr. Stephen also hired a live-in nanny.

6. Two years later, another woman was accepted. Thus, there were two women present when the residents went through their weekly sexual pantomime.

7. In a poster session, researchers do not deliver papers. Instead, they post information about each study (such as methods, research population, findings), and stand nearby so that meeting participants can question them. On occasion, researchers also distribute handouts describing the study.

8. The minor OR was used for small procedures that did not need the services of an anesthesiologist. As an experienced nurse-anesthetist, Dr. Stephen had far more knowledge and confidence than the "guys" in her ability to "sedate" patients so as to keep them comfortable while she operated.

9. Bates was paid for the research.

10. Of the twelve residents in the program, seven had scores that were higher than hers, and four had scores that were lower.

11. All the residents received the same letter, but she was the only one doing several research projects with him.

12. She said of this: "Dr. Bates could not *bear* to *acknowledge* that I had done the best in the program, in the ninetieth percentile, so he documented that I had gotten 76 percent, and that it was a forty-point change, which was not true. It was a 12 percent change in *score* and probably a forty-*percentile* change. So there was some ambiguity there. And I actually asked him to rewrite the letter with accurate numbers, which he did not do. I guess it was pretty ballsy to ask him to make it accurate."

13. The letter taking her off probation did not arrive until the last day of the term. Despite the fact that some of the male residents, who had been put on probation at the same time as Dr. Stephen, had lower scores on the fourth-year in-service exams than she, none needed a letter to get off probation. So far as she knew, the probation quietly evaporated for the men, allowing all of them to take the senior trip.

## 9. Surgeons in This Day and Age

1. The women residents at one training program schedule a weekly GNO (girls' night out), when they all dine together and chat, occasionally inviting a senior woman to come and talk to them. Such social bonding provides support, comfort, and advice. A group like this would have been far more difficult to establish in the Southern program where Dr. Stephen was trained; the senior men would have found such female bonding highly threatening, and would have used every weapon at their disposal, from threats to ridicule, to crush it. The difficulty in establishing such a GNO, however, probably indicates how helpful such female bonding would have been.

2. In 1917 a female professor of obstetrics and gynecology at the Woman's Medical College of Pennsylvania emphasized how important it is for women to incorporate surgical knowledge from other women: "The woman student sees women teaching and women doing the clinical work, women operating, and so on. Until I took my internship I had never seen a woman operate, and I do not think those of you who have had your training in this school can realize what it means never to have seen a woman doing that which to you seems second nature from your student days . . . It is almost inevitable, if you never have seen a woman doing anything, to think she cannot do it quite as well as a man, no matter how strongly you feel in favor of women" (Morantz-Sanchez: 255).

3. In 1996, of the thirty-three women I studied, fourteen were members of the Association of Women Surgeons (AWS). Of these fourteen, one was located through the AWS. Three of the thirty-three women practice in Canada; although the association has a few Canadian members, it is perhaps unfair to count them. What this means is that only thirteen of twenty-nine American women surgeons I studied (who were not located through the AWS) belonged to the organization (45 percent).

4. See Barinaga (1991); and *New York Times* June 4, 1991: A22.

5. E.g., Conley (1993).

6. See *The Making of a Surgeon,* by William Nolen (1970), for a description of the delights of becoming and being a surgeon in the Golden Age before government regulations, HMOs, and the growing distrust of patients curbed the surgeon's power and autonomy. Nolen's dedication reads: "My father was a lawyer. When I was a boy he

often said to me, 'Billy, if you're smart, when you grow up you'll be a doctor. Those bastards have it made.' I took my father's advice, and I dedicate this book to his memory." Throughout the book, it is obvious that Nolen feels that, as a surgeon, he *does* have it made. I discuss these issues in *Expected Miracles: Surgeons at Work*, in the chapter entitled "It's No Fun Anymore."

Was the Golden Age better? It depends on where one stands—or reclines—in relation to the operating table. Surely it was better for male surgeons, who were free to *tell*, not ask, patients what procedures would be performed, charge whatever the traffic would bear, and indulge in temper tantrums, hurling trays of instruments across the operating room to express rage or even pique. It was not better for women, who were excluded from surgery, except as nurses or patients. As for patients, I suspect that being operated on by a "godlike" surgeon, whose divinity and infallibility were acknowledged by surgeon and patient alike, may have had some benefits—but probably as many, if not more, drawbacks. The Golden Age was an age of charisma; today, charisma is distrusted, not honored.

7. I observed a woman surgeon teach an intern what to write on the chart of an elderly male patient. The patient had been discharged twice from the hospital to a rehabilitation facility, and each time he had returned he had been near death's door. The surgeon was now keeping him in the hospital, trying to get him in really good condition before discharging him. A rehab facility was so much cheaper, however, that Medicare kept disallowing the impoverished patient's hospital fees. She and the intern were consequently forced to make false notations on the patient's chart, reporting each day that his gangrenous leg looked worse. The devout Catholic surgeon was unhappy about lying and embarrassed at my hearing the conversation, but said that she was unable to figure out how to tell the truth and still get proper care for the old man.

8. Although I dislike the term "proletarianization," preferring Max Weber's phrase "the disenchantment of the world" (1958: 221) to describe bureaucratization and the "routinization of charisma," such developments could indeed be defined as proletarianization.

9. I still recall the tone of near-awe, indeed, almost love, used by my former husband when he spoke of his mentor and quoted his utterances. I have heard many older surgeons use this tone when speaking of their mentors.

10. An older surgeon told me how he liked to take promising young men under his wing: he would invite them to his home, and gently impart the social skills they may not have learned while growing up or during the grueling years of training (surgery can be a means of upward mobility for an intelligent and gifted student). Another surgeon described how he had stopped smoking when asked to do so by his mentor, despite the fact that he had previously ignored his parents' pleas to stop.

11. The HMO was started in the 1940s by an idealistic group who believed that doctors should *promote health* rather than treat illness. This nonprofit corporation signed contracts with unions and other companies to provide complete medical care for employees and their families. In the 1980s I spent time with an exemplary surgeon who worked for this HMO; convinced that this represented the future of medicine, he preferred being on salary so that he could give patients as much time and care as he thought necessary without worrying about costs (Cassell 1991: 98–100). Such HMOs are very different from today's for-profit corporations, which make money by driving out the competition and then delivering as little as possible at the highest possible price.

12. Insurance companies, hospitals, and Medicare have bureaucrats and/or committees to determine whether patients have been kept in the hospital longer than necessary. Since the decisionmakers—frequently nurses—know little about the individual patient (the decisions are made from charts) and are less highly trained than the doctors whose judgment they second-guess, their rulings are resented.

# REFERENCES

Abu-Lughod, Lila. 1990. "Can There Be a Feminist Ethnography?" *Women and Performance*, 5: 7–27.

———— 1993. *Writing Women's Worlds: Bedouin Stories*. Berkeley: University of California Press.

Adams, Abigail E. 1993. "Dyke to Dyke: Ritual Reproduction at a U.S. Men's Military College." *Anthropology Today*, 9 (5): 3–6.

Aisenberg, Nadya, and Mona Harrington. 1988. *Women of Academe: Outsiders in the Sacred Grove*. Amherst: University of Massachusetts Press.

Andrews, Edmund, M.D. 1861. "The Surgeon." *Chicago Medical Examiner*, 2: 587–598.

Barinaga, Marcia. 1991. "Sexism Charged by Stanford Physician." *Science*, 252 (June): 1484.

Bateson, Gregory. 1958. *Naven: A Survey of the Problems Suggested by a Composite Picture of the Culture of a New Guinea Tribe Drawn from Three Points of View*. Stanford, Calif.: Stanford University Press. Orig. pub. 1936.

Behar, Ruth. 1993. *Translated Woman: Crossing the Border with Esperanza's Story*. Boston: Beacon Press.

———— 1995. "Introduction: Out of Exile." In Ruth Behar and Deborah A. Gordon, eds., *Women Writing Culture*. Berkeley: University of California Press.

Belenky, Mary Field, B. Clinchy, N. Goldberger, and J. Tarule, eds. 1986. *Women's Ways of Knowing: The Development of Self, Voice and Mind*. New York: Basic Books.

Bonner, Thomas Neville. 1992. *To the Ends of the Earth: Women's Search for Education in Medicine.* Cambridge, Mass.: Harvard University Press.

Bordo, Susan. 1993. *Unbearable Weight: Feminism, Western Culture, and the Body.* Berkeley: University of California Press.

Bosk, Charles. 1976. *Forgive and Remember: Managing Medical Failure.* Chicago: University of Chicago Press.

Bourdieu, Pierre. 1977. *Outline of a Theory of Practice.* Trans. Richard Nice. Cambridge, England: Cambridge University Press. Orig. pub. 1972.

—— 1984. *Distinction: A Social Critique of the Judgement of Taste.* Trans. Richard Nice. Cambridge, Mass.: Harvard University Press. Orig. pub. 1979.

—— 1990a. *The Logic of Practice.* Trans. Richard Nice. Stanford, Calif.: Stanford University Press. Orig. pub. 1980.

—— 1990b. "Fieldwork in Philosophy." In Bourdieu, *In Other Words: Essays Towards a Reflexive Sociology.* Trans. Mathew Adamson. Stanford, Calif.: Stanford University Press.

"Breaking the Barrier." 1994. *New York Times,* November 2: A23.

Briggs, Jean. 1970. *Never in Anger.* Cambridge, Mass.: Harvard University Press.

Brodkey, Linda, and Michelle Fine. 1992. "Presence of Mind in the Absence of Body." In Michelle Fine, ed., *Disruptive Voices: The Possibilities of Feminist Research.* Ann Arbor: University of Michigan Press.

Brown, Karen McCarthy. 1991. *Mama Lola: A Vodou Priestess in Brooklyn.* Berkeley: University of California Press.

Campbell, Anne. 1993. *Men, Women, and Aggression.* New York: Basic Books.

Cassell, Eric J. 1991. *The Nature of Suffering and the Goals of Medicine.* New York: Oxford University Press.

Cassell, Joan. 1977a. *A Group Called Women: Sisterhood and Symbolism in the Feminist Movement.* New York: David McKay. Rpt. Prospect Heights, Ill.: Waveland Press, 1989.

—— 1977b. "The Relationship of Observer to Observed in Peer Group Research." *Human Organization,* 36 (4): 412–416.

—— 1978. "Advocacy versus Understanding in the Study of a Contemporary Social Movement." *Western Canadian Journal of Anthropology,* 3 (1): 38–46.

—— 1986. "Dismembering the Image of God: Surgeons, Wimps, Heroes and Miracles." *Anthropology Today,* 2 (2): 13–16.

—— 1987a. "Of Control, Certitude and the 'Paranoia' of Surgeons." *Culture, Medicine and Psychiatry,* 11 (2): 229–249.

—— 1987b. "The Good Surgeon." *International Journal of Moral and Social Studies,* 2 (2): 155–171.

—— 1987c. "'Oh No They're Not My Shoes!': Fieldwork in the Blue Mountains of Jamaica." In Joan Cassell, ed., *Children in the Field: Anthropological Experiences.* Philadelphia: Temple University Press.

—— 1989. "The Fellowship of Surgeons." *International Journal of Moral and Social Studies,* 4 (3): 195–212.

—— 1991. *Expected Miracles: Surgeons at Work.* Philadelphia: Temple University Press.

Cassell, Joan, and Sue-Ellen Jacobs, eds. 1987. *Handbook of Ethical Issues in Anthropology.* Washington, D.C.: American Anthropological Association.

Cassell, Joan, and Murray L. Wax, eds. 1980. *Ethical Problems of Fieldwork.* Special issue of *Social Problems,* 27 (3).

Chodorow, Nancy. 1978. *The Reproduction of Mothering: Psychoanalysis and the Sociology of Gender.* Berkeley: University of California Press.

Clifford, James. 1986. "Introduction: Partial Truths." In James Clifford and George E. Marcus, eds., *Writing Culture: The Poetics and Politics of Ethnography.* Berkeley: University of California Press.

Coltrane, Scott. 1989. "Household Labor and the Routine Production of Gender." *Social Problems,* 36 (5): 473–490.

Conley, Frances K. 1993. "Toward a More Perfect World: Eliminating Sexual Discrimination in Academic Medicine." *New England Journal of Medicine,* 328 (5): 351–352.

Cornum, Rhonda. 1996. "Soldiering: The Enemy Doesn't Care If You're Female." In Judith Hicks Stiehm, ed., *Women and the U.S. Military.* Philadelphia: Temple University Press.

Coser, Lewis. 1974. *Greedy Institutions: Patterns of Undivided Commitment.* New York: Free Press.

Csordas, Thomas J., ed. 1994. *Embodiment and Experience: The Existential Ground of Culture and Self.* New York: Cambridge University Press.

DeVault, Marjorie L. 1991. *Feeding the Family: The Social Organization of Caring as Gendered Work.* Chicago: University of Chicago Press.

Dumont, Jean Paul. 1978. *The Headman and I: Ambiguity and Ambivalence in the Fieldworking Experience.* Austin: University of Texas Press.

"Early Reports of Abuse Cited in Citadel Inquiry: Handling of Harassment Case Is Criticized." 1997. *New York Times,* January 22: A8.

Favret-Saada, Jeanne. 1980. *Deadly Words: Witchcraft in the Bocage*. Trans. C. Cullen. Cambridge, England: Cambridge University Press.

Fine, Michelle, ed. 1992. *Disruptive Voices: The Possibilities of Feminist Research*. Ann Arbor: University of Michigan Press.

Fine, Michelle, and Pat Macpherson. 1992. "Over Dinner: Feminism and Adolescent Female Bodies." In Michelle Fine, ed., *Disruptive Voices: The Possibilities of Feminist Research*. Ann Arbor: University of Michigan Press.

Finkler, Kaja. 1994. "Sacred Healing and Biomedicine Compared." *Medical Anthropology Quarterly*, 8 (2): 178–197.

Floge, Liliane, and Deborah Merrill. 1985. "Tokenism Reconsidered: Male Nurses and Female Physicians in a Hospital Setting. *Social Forces*, 64: 925–947.

Gatens, Moira. 1996. *Imaginary Bodies: Ethics, Power and Corporeality*. London: Routledge.

Geertz, Clifford. 1988. *Lives and Works: The Anthropologist as Author*. Stanford, Calif.: Stanford University Press.

Gilligan, Carol. 1982. *In a Different Voice: Psychological Theory and Women's Development*. Cambridge, Mass.: Harvard University Press.

Gillison, Gillian. 1993. *Between Culture and Fantasy: A New Guinea Highlands Mythology*. Chicago: University of Chicago Press.

Ginsburg, Faye, and Anna Lowenhaupt Tsing. 1990. "Introduction." In Ginsburg and Tsing, eds., *Uncertain Terms: Negotiating Gender in American Culture*. Boston: Beacon Press.

Ginsburg, Ruth Bader. 1993. "Concurrence to *Harris v. Forklift Systems, Inc.*" S10 US17, 25 (1993). Argued October 13, 1993. Decided November 9, 1993.

Goffman, Erving. 1967. "The Nature of Deference and Demeanor." In Goffman, *Interaction Ritual*. Garden City, N.Y.: Anchor Books.

Good, Byron J. 1994. *Medicine, Rationality and Experience: An Anthropological Perspective*. Cambridge: Cambridge University Press.

Good, Mary-Jo Delvecchio, Paul E. Brodwin, Byron J. Good, and Arthur Kleinman, eds. 1992. *Pain as Human Experience: An Anthropological Perspective*. Berkeley: University of California Press.

Gordon, Deborah A. 1988. "Writing Culture, Writing Feminism: The Poetics and Politics of Experimental Ethnography." *Inscriptions*, 3–4: 8–21.

Gordon, Deborah R. 1988a. "Clinical Science and Clinical Expertise: Changing Boundaries between Art and Science in Medicine." In

Margaret Lock and Deborah R. Gordon, eds., *Biomedicine Examined*. Dordrecht, Netherlands: Kluwer Academic Publishers.

—— 1988b. "Tenacious Assumptions in Western Medicine." In Margaret Lock and Deborah R. Gordon, eds., *Biomedicine Examined*. Dordrecht Netherlands: Kluwer Academic Publishers.

Gregor, Thomas. 1985. *Anxious Pleasures: The Sexual Lives of an Amazonian People*. Chicago: University of Chicago Press.

Hahn, Robert A., and Atwood D. Gaines. 1985. *Physicians of Western Medicine: Anthropological Approaches to Theory and Practice*. Dordrecht, Netherlands: D. Reidel.

Harding, Sandra. 1987. "Introduction: Is There a Feminist Methodology?" In Sandra Harding, ed., *Feminism and Methodology*. Bloomington: Indiana University Press.

Haraway, Donna J. 1991. "'Gender' for a Marxist Dictionary: The Sexual Politics of a Word." In Haraway, *Simians, Cyborgs, and Women: The Reinvention of Nature*. New York: Routledge, Chapman and Hall.

Herdt, Gilbert H. 1981. *Guardians of the Flutes: Idioms of Masculinity*. New York: Columbia University Press.

Hunter, Kathryn Montgomery. 1991. *Doctors' Stories: The Narrative Structure of Medical Knowledge*. Princeton: Princeton University Press.

Hymes, Dell, ed. 1969. *Reinventing Anthropology*. New York: Random House.

Jamieson, Kathleen Hall. 1995. *Beyond the Double Bind: Women and Leadership*. New York: Oxford University Press.

Kanter, Rosabeth Moss. 1977a. *Men and Women of the Corporation*. New York: Basic Books.

—— 1977b. "Some Effects of Proportions on Group Life: Skewed Sex Ratios and Responses to Token Women." *American Journal of Sociology*, 82: 985–990.

Kaprow, Miriam Lee. 1990. "Men's Studies, Male Firefighters." Paper presented at the fifth Congreso de Antropologia, Granada, Spain, December 11–14.

—— 1991. "Magical Work: Firefighters in New York." *Human Organization*, 50 (1): 97–103.

—— n.d. "Genteel Proletarianization: Regulating Leisure, Domesticating the Citizenry." Unpublished manuscript.

Katz, Pearl. 1981. "Ritual in the Operating Room." *Ethnology*, 20 (4): 335–350.

—— 1985. "How Surgeons Make Decisions." In Robert A. Hahn and

Atwood D. Gaines, eds., *Physicians of Western Medicine: Anthropological Approaches to Theory and Practice.* Dordrecht, Netherlands: D. Reidel.

Katz, Pearl, and Faris R. Kirkland. 1988. "Traditional Thought and Modern Western Surgery." *Social Science and Medicine,* 26 (12): 1175–1181.

Kemeny, M. Margaret. 1993. "Jonasson, Braunwald, and Morani: Three Firsts in American Surgery." *Archives of Surgery,* 128 (June): 644–645.

Kessler, Suzanne J., and Wendy McKenna. 1978. *Gender: An Ethnomethodological Approach.* New York: John Wiley and Sons.

Kinder, Barbara K. 1985. "Women and Men as Surgeons: Are the Problems Really Different?" *Current Surgery,* 42: 100–104.

Klass, Perri. 1987. *A Not Entirely Benign Procedure: Four Years as a Medical Student.* New York: New American Library.

———— 1988. "Are Women Better Doctors?" *New York Times Magazine,* April 10: 32–46.

Kleinman, Arthur. 1986. *Social Origins of Distress and Disease: Depression, Neurasthenia, and Pain in Modern China.* New Haven: Yale University Press.

———— 1988. *The Illness Narratives: Suffering, Healing, and the Human Condition.* New York: Basic Books.

———— 1995. *Writing at the Margin: Discourse between Anthropology and Medicine.* Berkeley: University of California Press.

Kondo, Dorinne K. 1990. *Crafting Selves: Power, Gender, and Discourses of Identity in a Japanese Workplace.* Chicago: University of Chicago Press.

Konner, Melvin. 1987. *Becoming a Doctor: A Journey of Initiation in Medical School.* New York: Penguin.

Kwakwa, Francis, and Olga Jonasson. 1996. "The Longitudinal Study of Surgical Residents, 1993 to 1994." *Journal of the American College of Surgeons,* 183 (5): 425–433.

Lavie, Smadar. 1990. *The Poetics of Military Occupation.* Berkeley: University of California Press.

Lichter, Linda S. 1994. "Home Truths." *Commentary,* 101 (June): 49–52.

Lock, Margaret, and Deborah Gordon, eds. 1988. *Biomedicine Examined.* Dordrecht Netherlands: Kluwer Academic Publishers.

Lorber, Judith. 1984. *Women Physicians: Careers, Status, and Power.* London: Tavistock.

———— 1985. "More Women Physicians: Will It Mean More Humane Health Care?" *Social Policy,* 15 (Summer): 50–54.

———— 1994. *Paradoxes of Gender.* New Haven: Yale University Press.

Luhrmann, Tanya M. 1994. "Increasing Embodiment: The Case of American Psychiatry." Paper presented at the annual meeting of the American Anthropological Association, December.

Lutkehaus, Nancy C. 1995. "Margaret Mead and the 'Rustling-of-the-Wind-in-the-Palm-Trees School' of Ethnographic Writing." In Ruth Behar and Deborah A. Gordon, eds., *Women Writing Culture.* Berkeley: University of California Press.

Lutz, Catherine. 1990. "The Erasure of Women's Writing in Sociocultural Anthropology." *American Ethnologist,* 17: 611–625.

——— 1995. "The Gender of Theory." In Ruth Behar and Deborah A. Gordon, eds., *Women Writing Culture.* Berkeley: University of California Press.

McDougall, Joyce. 1995. *The Many Faces of Eros.* New York: Norton.

Martin, Emily. 1987. *The Woman in the Body: A Cultural Analysis of Reproduction.* Boston: Beacon Press. Rpt. with new introduction 1992.

——— 1991. "The Ideology of Reproduction: The Reproduction of Ideology." In Faye Ginsburg and Anna Lowenhaupt Tsing, eds., *Uncertain Terms: Negotiating Gender in American Culture.* Boston: Beacon Press.

Martin, Jane Roland. 1994. "Methodological Essentialism, False Difference, and Other Dangerous Traps." *Signs: Journal of Women in Culture and Society,* 19 (3): 630–657.

Matsumoto, Valerie. 1996. "Reflections on Oral History: Research in a Japanese American Community." In Diane L. Wolf, ed., *Feminist Dilemmas in Fieldwork.* Boulder, Colo.: Westview.

McNamara, Jo Ann Kay. 1996. *Sisters in Arms: Catholic Nuns through Two Millennia.* Cambridge, Mass.: Harvard University Press.

Mead, Margaret. 1968. *Male and Female : A Study of the Sexes in a Changing World.* New York: Dell. Orig. pub. 1949.

Moir, Anne. 1991. *Brain Sex: The Real Difference between Men and Women.* New York: Carol Publishing.

Moore, Henrietta L. 1994. *A Passion for Difference: Essays in Anthropology and Gender.* Bloomington: Indiana University Press.

Morantz, Regina Markell. 1992. "Introduction: From Art to Science—Women Physicians in American Medicine, 1600–1980." In Regina Markell Morantz, Cynthia Stodola Pomerlau, and Carol Hansen Fenichel, eds., *In Her Own Words: Oral Histories of Women Physicians.* New Haven: Yale University Press.

Morantz-Sanchez, Regina Markell. 1985. *Sympathy and Science: Women Physicians in American Medicine.* New York: Oxford University Press.

Murphy, Yolanda, and Robert Murphy. 1974. *Women of the Forest*. New York: Columbia University Press.

Myerhoff, Barbara G. 1974. *Peyote Hunt: The Sacred Journey of the Huichol Indians*. Ithaca: Cornell University Press.

——— 1979. *Number Our Days*. New York: Simon and Schuster.

Nader, Laura. 1969. "Up the Anthropologist: Perspectives Gained from Studying Up." In Dell Hymes, ed., *Reinventing Anthropology*. New York: Random House.

Narayan, Kirin. 1989. *Storytellers, Saints and Scoundrels: Folk Narrative in Hindu Religious Teaching*. Philadelphia: University of Pennsylvania Press.

Noddings, Nell. 1984. *Caring: A Feminine Approach to Ethics and Moral Education*. Berkeley: University of California Press.

Nolen, William. 1970. *The Making of a Surgeon*. New York: Random House.

O'Neill, Molly. 1994. "A Surgeon's War on Breast Cancer: A Woman Full of Contradictions Is Both a Tough Fighter and a Gentle Healer." *New York Times*, June 29: C1.

Polanyi, Michael. 1967. *The Tacit Dimension*. Garden City, N.Y.: Doubleday Anchor.

Prell, Riv-Ellen. 1990. "Rage and Representation: Jewish Gender Stereotypes in American Culture." In Faye Ginsburg and Anna Lowenhaupt Tsing, eds., *Uncertain Terms: Negotiating Gender in American Culture*. Boston: Beacon Press.

Ramos, Sylvia M., and Cheryl J. Feiner. 1989. "Women Surgeons: A National Survey." *Journal of the American Medical Women's Association*, 44 (1): 21–25.

Rapp, Rayna. 1990. "Constructing Amniocentesis: Maternal and Medical Discourses." In Faye Ginsburg and Anna Lowenhaupt Tsing, eds., *Uncertain Terms: Negotiating Gender in American Culture*. Boston: Beacon Press.

Robbins, Derek. 1991. *The Work of Pierre Bourdieu*. Boulder, Colo.: Westview.

Rogers, Carla, Elizabeth Shakin Kunkel, and Howard L. Field. 1994. "Impact of Pregnancy during Training on a Psychiatric Resident Cohort." *Journal of the Medical Women's Association*, 49 (2): 49–52.

Rogers, Carolyn M., ed. 1995. *Socio-Economic Factbook for Surgery, 1995*. Chicago: American College of Surgeons.

Rosenthal, Elizabeth. 1997. "Older Doctors and Nurses See Jobs at Stake:

Big Paychecks Become Cost Cutters' Targets." *New York Times*, January 26: A1.

Ruddick, Sarah. 1989. *Maternal Thinking: Toward a Politics of Peace*. Boston: Beacon Press.

Said, Edward. 1978. *Orientalism*. New York: Pantheon.

Sheldon, George. 1996. "Editorial: The Longitudinal Study." *Journal of the American College of Surgeons*, 183 (5): 525–526.

Scheper-Hughes, Nancy, and Margaret M. Lock. 1987. "The Mindful Body: A Prolegomenon to Future Work in Medical Anthropology." *Medical Anthropology Quarterly*, 1 (1): 6–41.

Schmitt, Eric. 1994a. "Generals Oppose Combat by Women." *New York Times*, June 17: A1.

——— 1994b. "Pilot's Death Renews Debate over Women in Combat Role." *New York Times*, October 30: A33.

Shepherd, Naomi. 1993. *A Price below Rubies: Jewish Women as Rebels and Radicals*. Cambridge, Mass.: Harvard University Press.

Simmel, Georg. 1950. "Secrecy." In Simmel, *The Sociology of Georg Simmel*, ed. Kurt Wolff. Glencoe, Ill.: Free Press.

Smith, William C., Jr. 1996. *Report on Medical School Faculty Salaries, 1995–1996*. Washington, D.C.: Association of American Medical Colleges.

"Stanford Surgeon Quits, Citing Sex Harassment." 1991. *New York Times*, June 4: A22.

Starr, Paul. 1982. *The Social Transformation of American Medicine*. New York: Basic Books.

Stoller, Paul. 1989a. *The Taste of Ethnographic Things: The Senses in Anthropology*. Philadelphia: University of Pennsylvania Press.

——— 1989b. *Fusion of the Worlds: An Ethnography of Possession among the Songhay of Niger*. Chicago: University of Chicago Press.

Stoller, Paul, and Cheryl Olkes. 1987. *In Sorcery's Shadow: A Memoir of Apprenticeship among the Songhay of Niger*. Chicago: University of Chicago Press.

Tannen, Deborah. 1990. *You Just Don't Understand: Women and Men in Conversation*. New York: William Morrow.

——— 1994. *Talking from 9 to 5: How Women's and Men's Conversational Styles Affect Who Gets Heard, Who Gets Credit, and What Gets Done at Work*. New York: William Morrow.

Tedlock, Barbara. 1991. "From Participant Observation to the Observation of Participation: The Emergence of Narrative Ethnography." *Journal of Anthropological Research*, 47 (1): 69–94.

———— 1992. *The Beautiful and the Dangerous: Encounters with Zuni Indians.* New York: Penguin.

———— 1995. "Works and Wives." In Ruth Behar and Deborah A. Gordon, eds., *Women Writing Culture.* Berkeley: University of California Press.

Tiger, Lionel. 1970. *Men in Groups.* New York: Vintage.

Turner, Victor. 1967. "Lunda Medicine and the Treatment of Disease." In Turner, *The Forest of Symbols: Aspects of Ndembu Ritual.* Ithaca: Cornell University Press.

Unger, Rhoda K. 1989. *Representations: Social Constructions of Gender.* Amityville, N.Y.: Baywood.

Walsh, Elsa. 1995. *Divided Lives: The Public and Private Struggles of Three Accomplished Women.* New York: Simon and Schuster.

Wax, Murray L., and Joan Cassell, eds. 1989. *Federal Regulations: Ethical Issues and Social Research.* Boulder, Colo.: Westview.

Weber, Max. 1958. *The Protestant Ethic and the Spirit of Capitalism.* Trans. A. M. Henderson and Talcott Parsons. New York: Oxford University Press. Orig. pub. 1924.

West, Candace, and Sarah Fenstermaker. 1995. "Doing Difference." *Gender and Society,* 9: 8–37.

West, Candace, and Don H. Zimmerman. 1987. "Doing Gender." *Gender and Society,* 1 (2): 125–151.

"Why Would a Girl Go into Surgery?" 1986. *Journal of the American Medical Women's Association,* 41 (2): 59–60.

Wilson, Edward O. 1975. "Human Decency Is Animal." *New York Times Magazine,* October 12.

———— 1978. *On Human Nature.* Cambridge, Mass.: Harvard University Press.

Wolfe, Tom. 1979. *The Right Stuff.* New York: Random House.

# INDEX